WILDERNESS AND TRAVEL MEDICINE

A COMPLETE WILDERNESS MEDICINE AND TRAVEL MEDICINE HANDBOOK

SAM FURY

Illustrated by
NEIL GERMIO

Edited by
MAX JH POWERS

Copyright SF Nonfiction Books © 2015

Updated 2021 ©

www.SFNonfictionBooks.com

All Rights Reserved
No part of this document may be reproduced without written consent from the author.

WARNINGS AND DISCLAIMERS

The information in this publication is made public for reference only.

Neither the author, publisher, nor anyone else involved in the production of this publication is responsible for how the reader uses the information or the result of his/her actions.

CONTENTS

Introduction   xvii

Patient Care   1
First Aid Kit   2

PART ONE: MUST-READ INFORMATION

BASIC HUMAN ANATOMY

Circulatory System   9
Digestive System   10
Endocrine System   12
Immune System   15
Integumentary System   16
Genitourinary System   17
Musculoskeletal System   20
Nervous System   21
Respiratory System   23

PREVENTION

General Health and Fitness   27
Personal Hygiene   29
Vaccinations   34

MEDICATIONS GUIDE

Using the Medications Recommended in This Book   39
Alternative Remedies Vs Pharmaceuticals   41
General Safe Use Information for all Medications   42
Analgesics, Anti-Inflammatory Drugs, and Fever Reducers   44
Antibiotics   48
Anti-fungals   52

Antihistamines	54
Antiseptics	55
Antiviral Drugs	57
Haemostatics	58
High-Altitude Medications	59
Motion Sickness, Nausea, and Vomiting	60
Medicinal Plants	61
Miscellaneous	65

IMMEDIATE FIRST AID

CRITICAL FIRST AID

Assess the Situation	71
Mental Status: AVPU	72
Airway	74
Breathing	79
Circulation	80
Severe Bleeding	85
Nervous System	88
Anaphylaxis	89
Heart Attack	92
Pressure Immobilization Technique	93
Sucking Chest Wound	95
Mass Casualty Critical Assessment	96

SECONDARY EXAM

Recording Your Findings	101
Physical Exam	102
History	108
Vital Signs	109

OPEN WOUNDS, SKIN INFECTIONS, AND SEPSIS

Open Wounds	115
Impaling Objects	117
Skin Infection and Sepsis	118

MOVING A PATIENT

Drags	123
Carries	124

IMPROVISED LITTERS

Patient Packing	133
Non-Rigid Litters	134
Rigid Litters	136

PART TWO: DIAGNOSIS & TREATMENTS   141

ENVIRONMENTALLY INDUCED

ALTITUDE INDUCED

General Prevention of Altitude-Induced Illnesses	147
Acute Mountain Sickness (AMS)	148
HAPE and HACE	150
HAFE	152
High-Altitude Pharyngitis and Bronchitis	153
Peripheral Edema	154

ANIMALS: MARINE

GENERAL TREATMENTS

Marine Toxins	159
Spiny Injuries	160
Barracuda	161
Blue-Ringed Octopus	162
Bristle-Worm	164
Catfish	165
Conus	167
Coral	169
Jellyfish	171
Leeches	173
Moray Eel	175
Sea Cucumber	176
Sea Lion	177

Sea Snake	178
Sea Urchin	180
Sharks	182
Spine Fish	183
Sponges	185
Stingray	187
Weever Fish	189

ANIMALS: TERRESTRIAL

General Prevention of Animal Attack	193
Ant Bites	194
Bed Bugs	195
Bee/Wasp Sting	197
Caterpillars	198
Cat-Scratch Disease	200
Fleas	201
Insects: General	202
Mammalian Bites	204
Rabies	206
Mosquitoes	207
Dengue Fever	208
Japanese Encephalitis	209
Malaria	211
West Nile Virus	213
Yellow Fever	214
Cutaneous Myiasis	216
Mites and Chiggers	217
Porcupines	219
Scorpions	220
Snakes	221
Pressure-Immobilization Technique	223
Ticks	225
Lyme Disease	226
Rocky Mountain Spotted Fever	227

Tick Paralysis ... 228

LICE

Head Lice ... 231
Pubic Lice ... 233
Body Lice ... 234

COLD AND/OR WATER INDUCED

Cold Water Immersion ... 237
Drowning ... 240
Frostbite ... 242
Hypothermia ... 245
Saltwater Sores ... 248
Trench Foot ... 249

DIVING INDUCED

Alternobaric Vertigo ... 253
Arterial Gas Embolism ... 255
Contaminated Breathing Gas ... 256
Decompression Sickness ... 257
Inner Ear Barotrauma ... 259
Mask Squeeze ... 260
Nitrogen Narcosis ... 261
Hot Tub Folliculitis ... 262
Pulmonary Barotrauma ... 263
Sinus Squeeze ... 264
Tooth Squeeze ... 265

HEAT AND/OR SUN INDUCED

Burns ... 269
Heat Edema ... 273
Heat Exhaustion ... 274
Heat Rash ... 275
Heat Stroke ... 276
Heat Syncope ... 278
Hyponatremia ... 279

MISCELLANEOUS ENVIRONMENTAL ILLNESSES

Allergic Reactions	283
Hay Fever	285
Carbon Monoxide Poisoning	286
Jet Lag	288
Lightning	290
Radiation Sickness	293
Smoke Inhalation	297
Toxic Plants	299

HEAD

BRAIN

Acute Stress Reaction	305
Epidural Hematoma	306
Increasing Intracranial Pressure	307
Insomnia	309
Meningitis	311
Seizure	312
Stroke	314
Traumatic Brain Injury	316

HEADACHES AND MIGRAINES

Dehydration Headache	319
Sinus Headache	320
Tension Headache	321
Migraines	322

EARS

External Otitis	325
Otitis Media	327
Ear Wax	329
Foreign Bodies in the Ear	331
Perforated Eardrum	333

EYES

Eye Patching	337
Foreign Bodies in the Eye	338
Corneal Abrasion	339
Acute Angle-Closure Glaucoma	340
Conjunctivitis	341
Corneal Erosion	343
Corneal Ulcer	344
Displaced Contact Lens	345
Giant Cell Arteritis	346
Hyphema	347
Impaling Object in the Eye	348
Solar/Ultraviolet Keratitis	349
Stye	351

MOUTH AND TEETH

Toothache	355
Dental Extraction	357
Avulsion	360
Dry Socket	361
Aphthous Ulcers	362
Broken or Chipped Tooth	363
Cold Sores	364
Condensing Osteitis	365
Dental Abscess	366
Fractured Tooth	367
Gingivitis and Gum Disease	368
Lost Filling	369
Luxation	370
Mandibular Dislocation	371
Myofascial Dysfunction/Pain	372
Thrush	373
Tonsillitis	374

NOSE

Broken Nose	377
Foreign Body in the Nose	378
Nosebleed	379

| Raw Nose | 380 |
| Sinusitis | 381 |

CIRCULATORY SYSTEM

| Fainting | 385 |
| Internal Bleeding | 387 |

DEHYDRATION AND VOLUME SHOCK

Dehydration	391
Volume Shock	393
Rehydration Plan	394

DIABETES-RELATED ILLNESSES

| Hypoglycemia | 397 |
| Hyperglycemia | 398 |

DIGESTIVE SYSTEM

Abdominal Pain	401
Alcohol Poisoning	403
Hangovers	404
Appendicitis	406
Constipation	408
Diverticulitis	409
Food Poisoning	410
Gas	412
Heartburn	413
Hemorrhoids	414
Hepatitis	416
Nausea and Vomiting	418
Peptic Ulcer	419
Worms	420

DIARRHEA

| More Serious than Diarrhea | 423 |
| Dysentery | 425 |

SALMONELLA

Typhoid/Paratyphoid Fever   429

GENITOURINARY SYSTEM

Kidney Infection   433
Kidney Stones   434
Prostatitis   435
Urinary Tract Infections   436

VAGINAL INFECTIONS

Bacterial Vaginosis   441

PREGNANCY-RELATATED CONDITIONS

Delivery   445
Hyperemesis Gravidarum   446
Miscarriage   447
Pregnancy-Induced Hypertension   448
Tubal Pregnancy   449

SEXUALLY TRANSMITTED INFECTIONS

Chlamydia   453
Genital Herpes   455
Gonorrhea   457
Pelvic Inflammatory Disease   459

INTEGUMENTARY SYSTEM

Abscesses   463
Acne   465
Blisters and Hot Spots   466
Bruises   468
Chickenpox   469
Eczema   471
Shingles   472

Splinters	473
Fishhooks	475
Tinea/Ringworm	476
Athlete's Foot	477

NAIL INJURIES

Nail Avulsion	481
Ingrown Toenail	482
Crush Injuries	484

MUSCULOSKELETAL SYSTEM

Musculoskeletal Injuries in General	487
Immobilization	490
Amputations	495
Backache	497
Pneumothorax	498
Tetanus	500

DISLOCATIONS

Reductions	503

FRACTURES

Fractured Ribs	511
Flail Chest	512
Fractured Pelvis	513

SPRAINS AND STRAINS

Sprains	517
Strains	518

RESPIRATORY SYSTEM

Asthma	521
Bronchitis	525
Cold and Flu	527
Dry Cough	530

Pneumonia 531
Sore Throat 533
Strep Throat 534
Whooping Cough 535

References 538

Author Recommendations 539
About Sam Fury 541

THANKS FOR YOUR PURCHASE

Did you know you can get FREE chapters of any SF Nonfiction Book you want?

https://offers.SFNonfictionBooks.com/Free-Chapters

You will also be among the first to know of FREE review copies, discount offers, bonus content, and more.

Go to:

https://offers.SFNonfictionBooks.com/Free-Chapters

Thanks again for your support.

INTRODUCTION

This book is a comprehensive guide to wilderness and travel medicine. It started out as a personal reference that I could store on my phone while traveling.

Of course, there are many similar books, but I purposefully organized this one in a specific way for easy reference. Also, it contains information on what you can use when pharmaceuticals are not available. This is good for WSHTF scenarios or in foreign countries where you may have to improvise.

I want to stress that this is NOT a replacement for professional training or a doctor's advice. It is a reference manual and nothing more.

Enhanced Learning

Although this book is jam-packed with information covering a wide variety of field-treatable ailments, no amount of reading can compare to a practical-based medical course taught by a professional medical trainer. A standard first aid course is good, but a wilderness first aid course or higher is better.

How to Use This Book

The information in this book is very multifaceted. Many chapters refer to one another, and these are indicated in the text as "Related Chapters."

This book is comprised of two parts:

1. Must Read Information

The first part contains all the background knowledge needed to effectively use the information in this book. It covers the following:

Anatomy. A basic rundown of how the body's systems work individually and as a whole.

Prevention Medicine. How to avoid getting sick and/or injured in the first place.

Medications Guide. Important information on the safe use of the medications referenced in this book.

Immediate First Aid. Contains the information needed on what to do medically in urgent, life-threatening situations.

Secondary Exam. A secondary exam will help you to make an accurate medical diagnosis.

Moving a Patient. Learn a variety of methods to safely move a patient.

2. Diagnosis and Treatments

This section of the book contains all the information you need to diagnose and treat specific medical problems that are not covered in the Immediate First Aid chapter.

Information for each condition contains:

- A brief description of the condition.
- Symptoms that may be experienced as a result of the condition.
- Appropriate treatment(s) for the condition depending on the situation.
- Other supplementary information—e.g., causes, prevention, alternative remedies, and possible complications—may also be included where applicable.

Note: Depending on your situation, many of the treatments may not be viable. Innovate and do the best you can with what you have.

PATIENT CARE

Most of the treatments in this book are described as self-aid, but they can also be used to treat others.

It is important to remember that although you may be trying to help someone, it is ultimately up to them—or an advocate acting on their behalf—as to whether and how you can treat them. If they refuse or object to your help, you should respect their request.

It is also important to explain to patients the full range of options and let them choose which course of action to take. You can give them your recommendations, but it is up to them to make the final choice.

If a patient is medically incompetent or unable to give consent and there is no advocate, whether or not to help them is a decision you will have to make.

FIRST AID KIT

A basic first aid kit is something every traveler should carry. Exactly what you carry in it is dependent on your skills. Also consider if you will want to take it on board a plane since there are some items that will not be allowed.

Here is a sample first aid kit which is safe to have as carry-on luggage as long as the liquids do not exceed the 100-ml limit.

Since most travelers prefer to limit the amount of luggage they have, this sample kit is very minimalist, which means many things will have to be improvised if needed.

Further information about specific items and their use can be found in later chapters.

- Adhesive bandages: an assortment of sizes
- Amoxicillin/clavulanate, e.g., Augmentin (antibiotic)
- Anti-diarrheal, e.g., Imodium
- Aspirin (analgesic, anti-inflammatory)
- Ciprofloxacin, e.g., Cipro (antibiotic)
- Cloth tape
- Doxycycline, e.g., Vibramycin (antibiotic)
- Diphenhydramine, e.g., Benadryl (antihistamine)
- Gauze pads: Preferably sterile
- Gloves: Preferably non-latex
- Haemostatic, e.g., QuikClot (blood clotting agent)
- Hydrocodene (analgesic, strong)
- Laxative: preferably natural, e.g., Metamucil
- Lip balm
- SOAP notes and pencil
- Scissors: May not be able to take on board a plane, but if they are small enough, they should pass.
- Sunscreen: SPF 30 at a minimum
- Tick/splinter kit: Should include small tweezers and mini magnifying glass.

- Medications pertinent to your travels, e.g., high-altitude, SCUBA
- Personal medications, e.g., allergy/anaphylaxis, asthma, contact lenses

Also consider:

- Albuterol, even if non-asthmatic.
- Alternate antibiotics in case of allergy or other complication, e.g., pregnancy.
- Blister bandages.
- Epinephrine auto-injector, e.g., EpiPen, even if no known history of anaphylaxis.
- Eye wash, eye drops, and/or antibiotic eye drops.
- Oral thermometer.
- Roller bandage.
- Small LED flashlight.
- Triangular bandage(s).
- Vet wrap.
- Paperwork, e.g., notes from doctor for prescription drugs, first aid notes, inventory, etc.

If you do not trust natural remedies for certain (or all) things, then consider also including:

- Acetaminophen (analgesic).
- Antacid.
- Antifungal.
- Antiseptic.
- Burn gel.
- Decongestant.
- Dramamine (motion sickness).
- Hand sanitizer.
- Ibuprofen (analgesic, anti-inflammatory).
- Itch relief.
- Insect repellant: DEET 30% maximum or Picaridin.

- Triple antibiotic ointment.

Important Notes:

- Check your first aid kit regularly for expiration dates and refill any supplies that have been used.
- Please read the medications guide chapter before considering the use of any type of medication.
- Doctor notes for prescription drugs are recommended.

Related Chapters

- Must Read > Medications Guide
- Must Read > Secondary Exam

PART ONE: MUST-READ INFORMATION

BASIC HUMAN ANATOMY

The human body is truly amazing, but it does have its vulnerabilities. Everyone should take the time to learn about the human body in general as well as what it can and can't do.

A general overview of the body's main systems and how they work together will help with correct diagnoses and treatments. The body's systems will also be used in categorizing specific diagnoses and treatments within this book.

CIRCULATORY SYSTEM

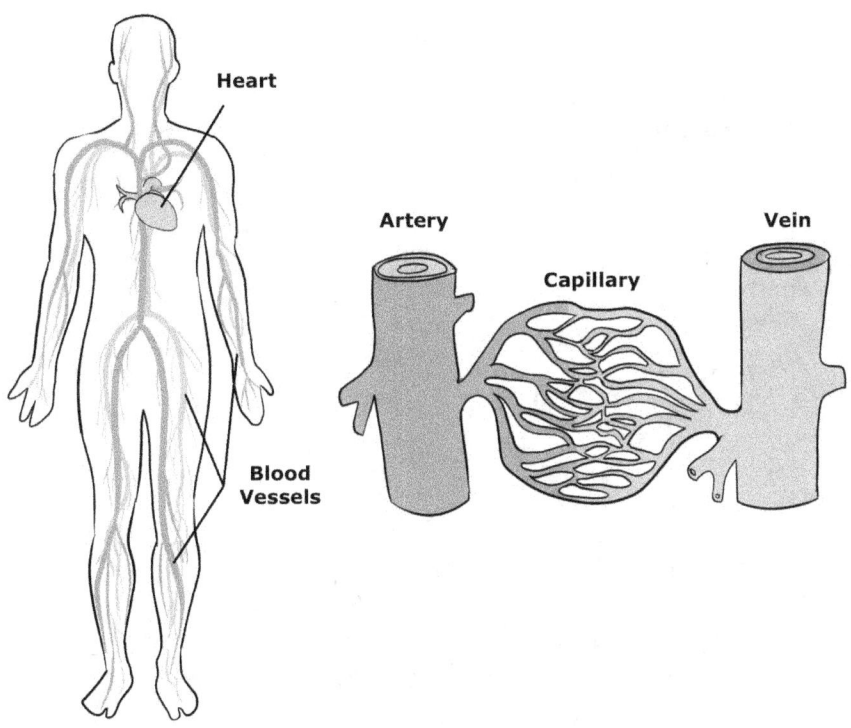

The circulatory (cardiovascular) system is made up of the heart and blood vessels (arteries, veins, and capillaries). The heart is like a pump which circulates blood to all the different parts of the body via the blood vessels.

Blood carries oxygen, nutrients, hormones, waste products, etc.

DIGESTIVE SYSTEM

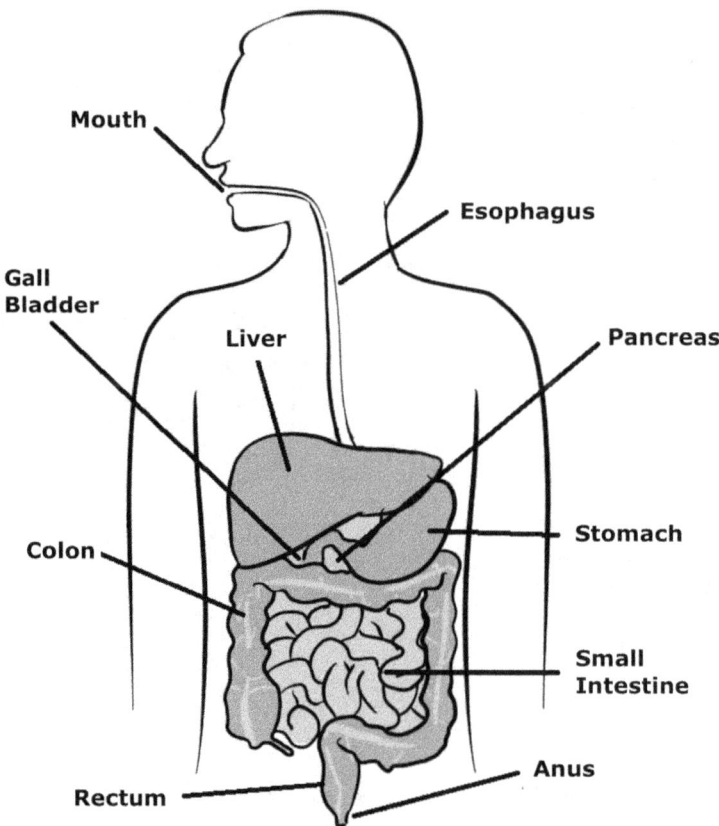

The main job of the digestive system is to break down food and convert it into nutritional molecules. These molecules are distributed throughout the body via the circulatory system. The digestive system also gets rid of everything that is unused in the form of excrement.

When a bite of food is taken, it marks the beginning of the digestive process. Through chewing and the mixture of saliva, the food is broken down into easily digested pieces. The food is then passed through the throat (larynx) and swallowed down the esophagus into the stomach.

The stomach adds acid and enzymes to the food while mixing and grinding it into a paste-like substance. Next is the small intestine, which uses enzymes from the pancreas and bile from the liver, as well as some help from the gallbladder (the gallbladder concentrates the bile from the liver, mainly by removing the water) to further break down the food and absorb nutrients into the blood stream.

Whatever is left over is then passed to the colon (large intestine). Water is removed, leaving behind mostly food debris and bacteria, i.e., feces. The feces (stool) are stored in a part of the colon called the sigmoid colon. Once the sigmoid colon is full, it is emptied into the rectum. The rectum holds the feces until it is told by the brain that it is okay to empty it. When it is time, the anal sphincters are relaxed and the feces is expelled.

ENDOCRINE SYSTEM

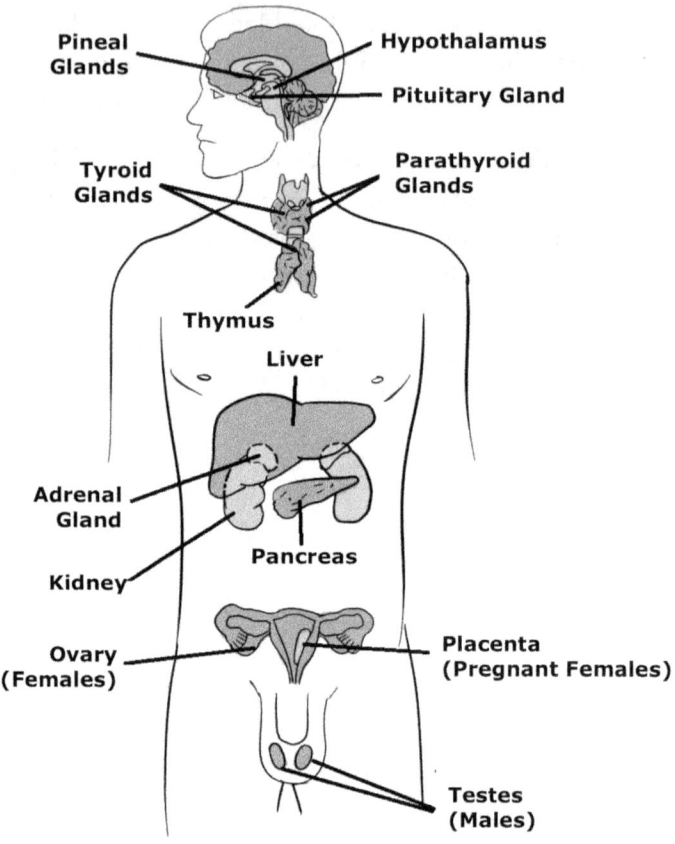

The endocrine system is the main system that coordinates the chemicals within the body. Hormones carry the body's chemical messages around the body. A gland is a group of cells that produces and secrete these chemicals.

Although nearly all organs and tissues produce their respective systems' endocrine hormones, the principal endocrine glands are the adrenal, parathyroid, pituitary, and thyroid glands, as well as the gonads and pancreas.

PART ONE: MUST-READ INFORMATION

The hypothalamus is a bunch of cells in the lower brain. The brain uses the hypothalamus to communicate with the pituitary gland.

At the base of the brain, just below the hypothalamus, is the pituitary gland. The pituitary gland is made up of two parts: the anterior lobe and the posterior lobe. The anterior lobe produces corticotrophin (stimulates the adrenal gland), growth hormones, prolactin (regulates milk production in mothers), and thyrotropin (stimulates the thyroid gland). It also releases endorphins to the nervous system which decrease feelings of pain, release the hormones which tell the sexual organs to produce sexual hormones, and control ovulation and menstruation in females.

The posterior lobe releases anti-diuretic hormones which help with the balance of water in the body as well as producing oxytocin which triggers uterine contractions during childbirth.

The two adrenal glands also have two parts. The outer part is the adrenal cortex, which produces corticosteroid hormones. The corticosteroid hormones regulate the immune system, metabolism, stress response, sexual development, sexual function, and salt-water balance.

The inner part of the adrenal gland is the adrenal medulla: it produces adrenaline (epinephrine). Epinephrine increases blood pressure and heart rate when the body experiences stress.

The gonads are the main source of sexual hormones. In men, they are the testes, which release androgens such as testosterone. Testosterone regulates puberty in adolescent males and helps communicate to the body when to produce more sperm. In females, the gonads are the ovaries, which produce eggs and release estrogen and progesterone. Estrogen regulates puberty, and both hormones regulate the menstrual cycle and help in pregnancy.

The pancreas produces insulin and glucagon which work together to maintain a steady level of glucose in the blood and keep the body supplied with fuel for creating and storing energy.

The pineal gland is in the brain; it secretes melatonin, which is believed to regulate sleeping patterns.

The thyroid produces the hormones that control the rate at which cells burn fuel from food to produce energy. The more of these hormones there are, the faster the chemical reactions in the body occur.

Attached to the thyroid are the parathyroids, which release the parathyroid hormone. The parathyroid hormone helps to regulate calcium in the blood.

IMMUNE SYSTEM

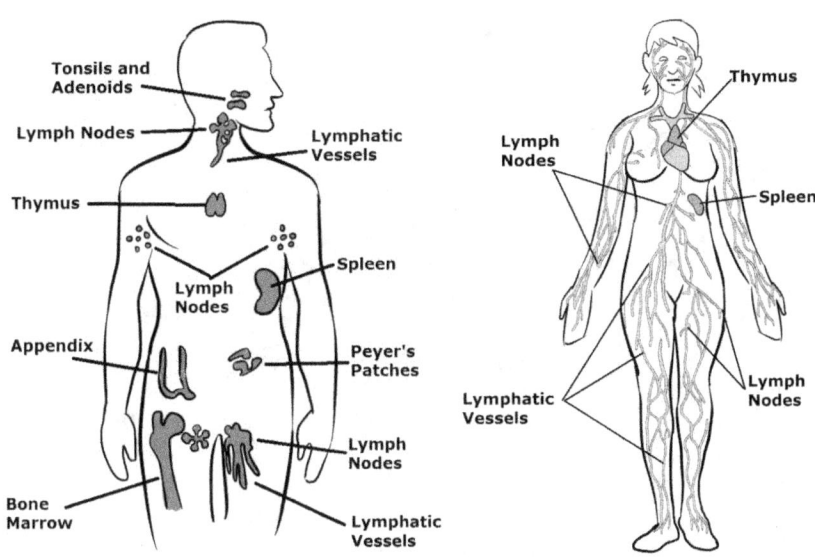

The immune system helps to protect the body from disease. It identifies pathogens (e.g., viruses), distinguishes them from healthy tissue, and then fights them.

It uses white blood cells (leukocytes) to combat the invaders. These white blood cells are produced and stored in the lymphoid organs such as bone marrow, the spleen, and the thymus. They are also stored around the body in the lymph nodes and other lymphoid tissue.

The leukocytes are transported around the body via the lymphatic vessels and blood vessels.

INTEGUMENTARY SYSTEM

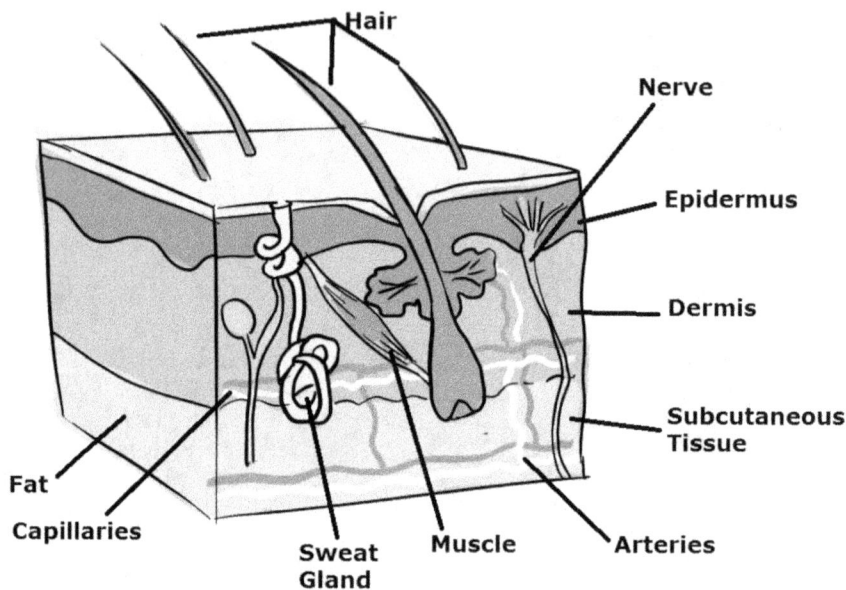

This is everything that covers the outside of the body including hair, nails, skin, sweat glands, etc.

This system protects the body from the outside world (e.g., infections, temperature), collects information via the skin (e.g., pain, temperature), helps regulate body temperature (e.g., capillary contraction, sweating), and stores water and fat.

GENITOURINARY SYSTEM

The genitourinary system includes the reproductive and urinary systems.

Urinary System

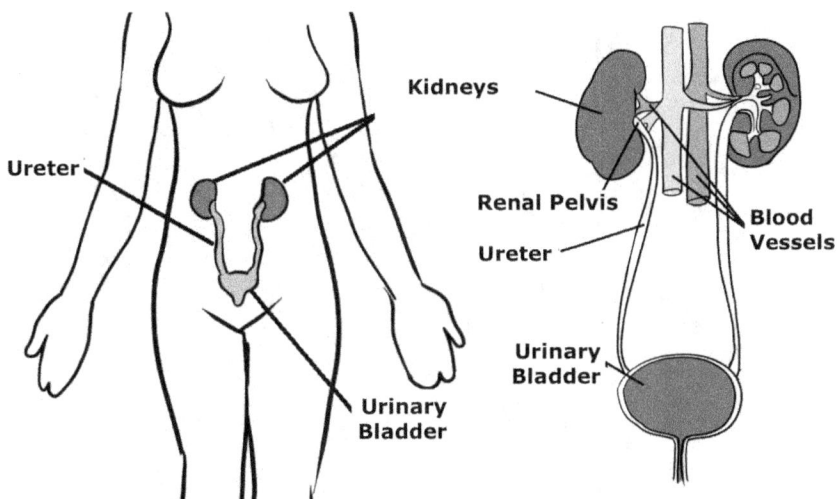

The main function of the urinary (renal) system is to expel excess ions, waste molecules, and water from the blood through urine. It also regulates blood pressure, blood volume, blood PH, electrolyte levels, and metabolite levels.

Blood is carried into the kidneys. The kidneys filter the waste and pass it to the bladder via the ureters. The urine is stored in the bladder until the time of urination. At that time, it passes through the urethra to the outside of the body.

Reproductive System

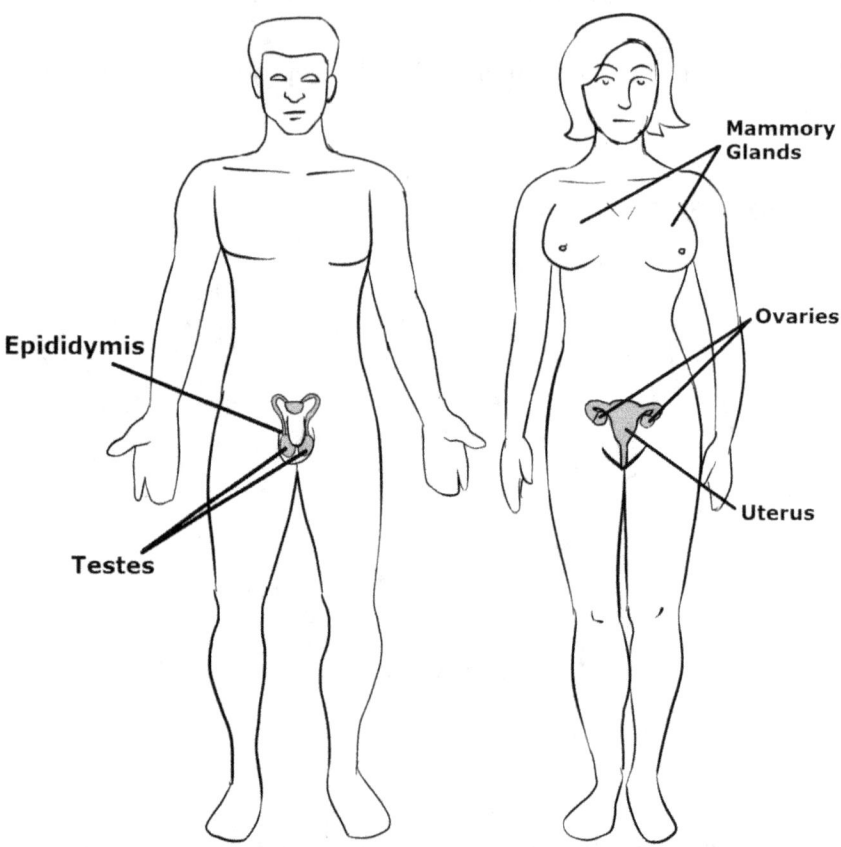

The reproductive system enables us to reproduce. It produces sperm in males and eggs in females. It also facilitates the joining of eggs and sperm in order to create a new organism, and it provides a place for the new organism to grow.

Male Reproductive System

The scrotum acts like a climate control facility for the testes. The testes, which are inside the scrotum, create testosterone and sperm. Once the sperm is made, it is stored in the epididymis where it matures until it is capable of fertilization.

When a man is sexually aroused, the sperm is passed into the vas deferens, which transports the mature sperm to the urethra via the ejaculatory ducts. During this phase of erection, urine is blocked from the urethra.

Throughout this process, the sperm is combined with other fluids to make up semen, neutralize traces of urine, and add fructose. This is done with the help of the seminal vesicles, the prostate gland, and the bulbourethral gland. At the time of orgasm, the semen is passed out through the penis.

Female Reproductive System

The ova (eggs) are produced in the ovaries. The ova are transported to the fallopian tube where they may be fertilized by the sperm. Once fertilized, the egg moves in the uterus and sticks to the uterine lining so it can mature.

If there is no fertilization, the uterine lining is discarded (menstrual flow).

As women get older, the female reproductive system stops making the female hormones needed for the reproduction system to work. This is called menopause.

MUSCULOSKELETAL SYSTEM

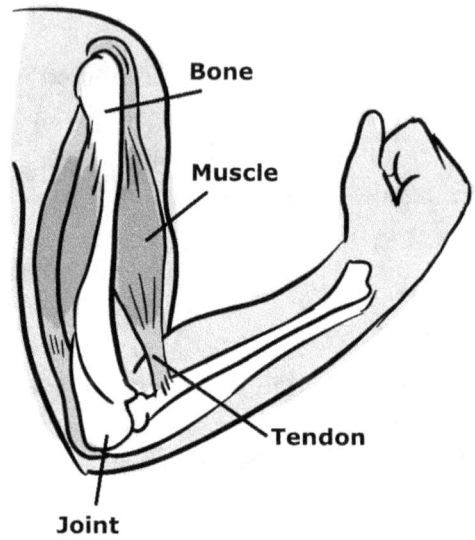

The musculoskeletal system is made up of the muscular system and the skeletal system. It includes all bones, cartilage, tendons, muscles, and ligaments. It gives us the ability to move and creates our basic body structure.

The larger bones also produce blood cells in the bone marrow, and all bones store phosphate and calcium.

NERVOUS SYSTEM

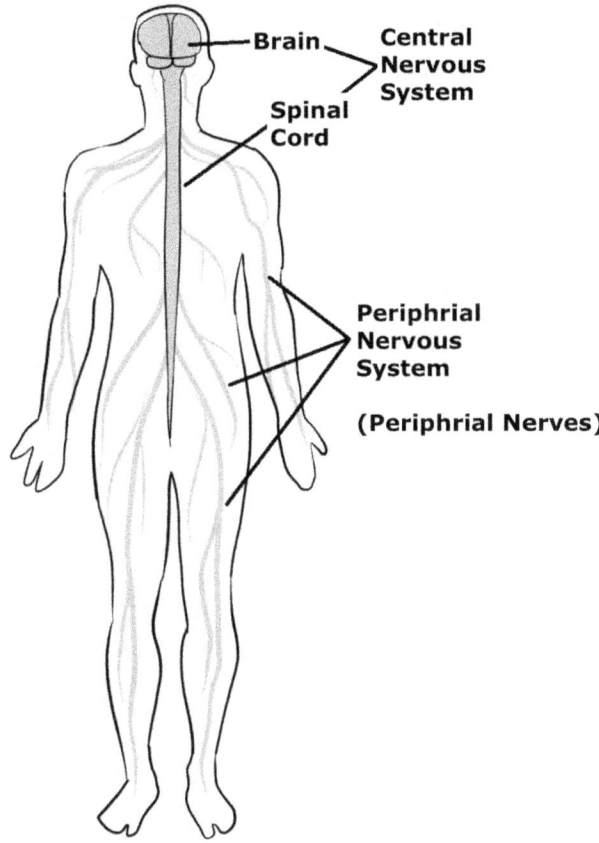

The nervous system is made up of the central nervous system and the peripheral nervous system. Together they use about 100 billion neurons which communicate with each other via electrical signals.

The central nervous system is made up of the brain and spinal cord. The peripheral nervous system includes all the nerves and neuron clusters (ganglia) in the rest of the body.

The peripheral nervous system collects information from all areas of the body (joints, muscles, skin, etc.) and sends it to the brain via the spinal cord. The brain collects information from the ears, eyes, mouth, and nose. It analyses all this information, performs all the important functions of the brain (e.g., memory, thinking, planning), and then sends out the instructions to the body via the nervous system.

RESPIRATORY SYSTEM

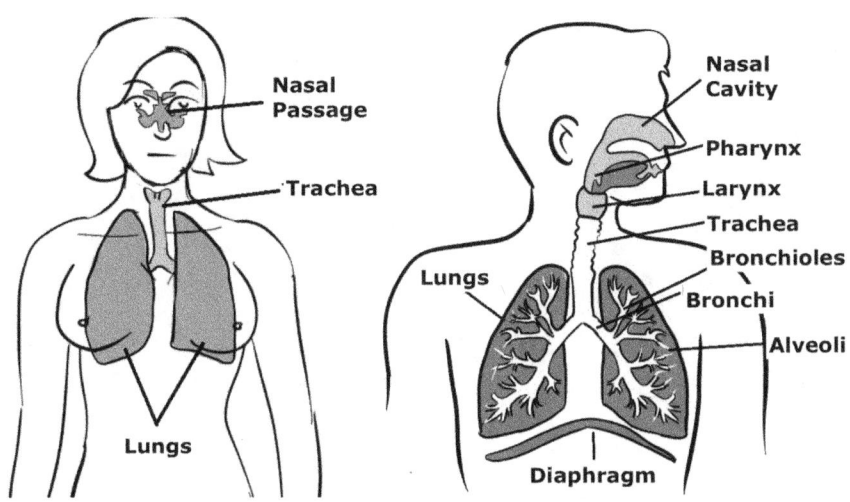

This is the system that enables us to breathe. It takes in oxygen from the air and expels water and carbon dioxide from the body.

Air gets breathed in and out via the mouth or nose. Inhaled air passes through the pharynx (throat) through the larynx (voice-box) and then to the trachea (windpipe). The air then gets passed to the bronchi, which split like tree branches into the lungs. The bronchi continue to split and get smaller and smaller, turning into bronchioles and, finally, into tiny sacs called the alveoli. Inside the alveoli, gas is exchanged with the blood cells in the capillaries. The main gases exchanged are oxygen (used by the body's cells) and carbon dioxide (expelled as a waste product).

The lungs are surrounded by muscles including the diaphragm and intercostal muscles, which work together like a pump to expand and compress the lungs, i.e., allowing air to be inhaled and exhaled.

PREVENTION

The best cure is always prevention.

Many injuries can be easily avoided, e.g., by not playing with wild animals, using sunscreen, warming up before exercise, watching where you are going, and wearing protective clothing.

Preventing illness is a matter of keeping in good health, and good health is basically comprised of four things: nutrition, exercise, recharging, and hygiene.

GENERAL HEALTH AND FITNESS

Nutrition

Nutrition is everything that you put into your body. Here are some guidelines to follow:

- Avoid unnecessary drugs (including alcohol, cigarettes, and overuse of pharmaceuticals) and excess fat, salt, and sugar.
- Eat a diet high in fruits, vegetables, and legumes.
- Detoxify your body every month or two. A simple way to do this is to consume nothing but water for 24 hours.
- Drink at least one liter of water a day, preferably two, and even more when exercising. Even better than water is green tea (it's packed with anti-oxidants).
- Eat a varied diet.
- Everything in moderation.
- Consider taking an immune system-boosting supplement and/or other multivitamin every other day, especially when traveling.
- In everyday life, use more garlic, ginger, chili, and raw honey in your cooking; apart from adding flavor, these are jam packed with 'anti-everything' properties.

In a survival situation, a common plant filled with vitamins and minerals is plantain. Make a tea out of it. Also, do not avoid sugar, salts, and fats. These are the nutrients that keep the body running, and you need all the nutrition you can get. It is only in modern life that we get far too much of them—everything in moderation.

Exercise

Exercise is any physical activity you do which results in an increased heart rate. Here are some guidelines to follow:

- Exercise regularly. As little as twenty minutes of focused exercise a day is enough.
- Stretch every day.

If you are in a survival situation, you may want to conserve energy. Survival activities will probably prove to be enough to keep fit (e.g., hunting).

Yoga is highly recommended and is referred to in some of the treatments in this book.

Recharging

Recharging refers to allowing your body and mind to recuperate.

Get enough rest (i.e., sleep) at least 6 hours a day, preferably 7 to 9.

Lower your stress levels. Things like aromatherapy, massages, meditation, and relaxing baths can all help to lower stress.

PERSONAL HYGIENE

Good nutrition, exercise, and recharging work together to keep your body strong to fight infections and injury. Good personal hygiene will help to stop infections from entering your body in the first place.

When traveling to unfamiliar places, you will be exposed to things your body has probably not encountered before. Your immune system will not be built up enough to combat these things, so personal hygiene becomes even more important.

Everything your mother told you to do as a child (e.g., washing your hands after using the bathroom or cleaning eating utensils after each use) you should do religiously when in an unfamiliar environment, especially if your travels lead you into a survival and/or wilderness situation. Even seemingly small things can turn disastrously bad.

Here is a daily hygiene routine you can follow in the case of a survival situation.

Start from the top of your body and work your way down, i.e., from head to toes. This is an example routine aimed at the worst possible scenario, i.e., a survival/collapsed society situation. You may not have to be so strict.

Keep as dry and clean as possible.

Wash every part of your body, preferably with soap. Drinking water is always the priority, so make the best with what you have.

Head

Shorter hair is always easier to keep clean.

Teeth

If the water is available, rinse your mouth out first thing in the morning and after every meal.

Dental Floss: Thin string-like substances can be used as dental floss, e.g., para-cord inner core, fishing line, or plant fiber (as long as the plant is safe). Tie an overhand knot in it to remove any difficult objects.

Mouthwash: A solution made of water and 1 to 3% hydrogen peroxide or clove oil will make a good mouthwash alternative. Beware that too much hydrogen peroxide or clove oil can burn your mouth.

If clove oil or hydrogen peroxide is not available, simple salt water is better than nothing. These alternative mouthwashes are also good to use as toothpaste if there is nothing else.

Toothbrush: A hardwood twig (live wood) that you have frayed by chewing can be used as a makeshift toothbrush. A piece of cloth could also be used. Even just your finger is better than nothing. It is also important to brush your gums. If your toothbrush is too harsh, use your finger.

Toothpaste: Baking soda makes good alternative toothpaste.

Body

Wash your entire body and check for parasites (lice, fleas, ticks, etc.), especially in hairy and moist areas (e.g., groin, armpits). Be careful not to crush any that you find. Pick them off.

Hands

Wash your hands before handling food or water that you are going to consume. If no disinfectant is available, just using running water is much better than nothing—the stronger the water pressure the better.

Whether you have soap, hand sanitizer, or just water, make sure you wash your hands properly. It should take about a minute to clean and dry them.

Get into all the nooks and crannies, e.g., between fingers and under fingernails.

Nails

Do your best to keep your nails clean, especially if you get a cut underneath them. Cut them if possible, but be careful not to over-cut them as that may lead to ingrown nails and/or infection.

Feet

Your feet are extremely important. You must keep them protected from injury. Wash, dry, and massage them regularly. Likewise, change and wash your socks regularly.

When hiking, check your feet often for blisters and/or hot spots. Take preventative measures.

Clothing

Keeping covered will protect you from the elements and insects.

Wash your clothes regularly for hygiene, as well as to make them last longer.

If no insect repellents are available, you can use smoke to fumigate them.

Minimize your exposure to mosquitoes.

Waste Management

Defecate in a designated spot at least 50 m away from your water and also away (preferably downwind) from camp. Make it out of the way but not inconvenient. You want to be able to get to it at night if needed.

After defecating, cover the feces with earth.

Drinking Water

Establish a drinking water collection point and ensure no one washes upstream from it. Downstream from the drinking water, choose a point for washing your body and clothes, and downstream from that, choose a point for washing dishes.

All water from natural and other questionable sources should be purified. Boiling it for 5 minutes is best, but bleach, iodine, and UV light (e.g., Steripens) also work.

Caring for the Sick

When caring for, or in the presence of, a sick person:

- Wash hands before and after contact.
- Wear a mask.
- Wear gloves.
- Wash down all possibly contaminated surfaces with disinfectant, e.g., diluted bleach.

The sick person should:

- Cover their mouth and nose with tissues when coughing, sneezing, etc.
- Dispose of tissues correctly (e.g., in the trash).
- Keep their distance from others, at least 150 cm.
- Be quarantined if a high fever is present.

Soap Making

White ashes, sand, loamy soil (a mixture of sand, clay, silt, and organic matter) and even some plants can be used as alternative soaps.

You can make soap by mixing animal fat or vegetable oil with alkali, and alkali can be produced from wood or seaweed ash:

- Wash the ash with water.
- Strain and then boil it with the oil or animal fat.
- Once it is boiling, bring it down to a simmer to burn off all the liquid.
- Adding pine resin, clove oil, etc., will give it antiseptic properties.
- Let it cool before using.

Note: Too much alkali will dry your skin.

Related Chapters

- Diagnosis and Treatments > Integumentary System > Blisters and Hot Spots
- Diagnosis and Treatments > Environmentally Induced

VACCINATIONS

The following vaccinations are recommended for world travelers by the World Health Organization. They are accurate at the time of this writing.

It is a good idea to have all your vaccinations recorded in the World Health Organization (WHO) International Certificate of Vaccination:

Who.int/ihr/IVC200_06_26.pdf?ua=1

Routine Vaccinations

These are vaccinations that everyone should have:

- Diphtheria, tetanus, and pertussis
- Hepatitis B (Hep B)
- Haemophilus influenzae type B
- Human papillomavirus
- Influenza
- Measles, mumps, and rubella
- Pneumococcal
- Polio
- Rotavirus
- Tuberculosis (BCG)
- Varicella

Selective Vaccinations

These are vaccines that you should have if intending to go to high-risk areas:

- Hepatitis A
- Cholera
- Japanese encephalitis

- Meningococcal
- Rabies
- Tick-borne encephalitis
- Typhoid fever
- Yellow fever

Required Vaccinations

These are vaccines that you are required to have if entering certain countries:

- Yellow fever
- Meningococcal
- Polio

Check for latest information on required vaccines at WHO.int/wer/en.

MEDICATIONS GUIDE

This chapter lists most of the medications referred to in this book, both natural and pharmaceutical. It includes common names (in parenthesis), important notes, and veterinary substitutes if applicable.

Veterinary substitutes are given because they are available without a prescription and they also may be the only option available in certain circumstances. Only use veterinary substitutes as a very last resort.

USING THE MEDICATIONS RECOMMENDED IN THIS BOOK

Brand names for drugs are given in parenthesis, but that does not mean that there are no other brands available.

Information presented here is by no means thorough, e.g., there are many unmentioned cautions and side effects.

Medications that are not listed in the treatments might still be effective, e.g., analgesics for general pain relief.

Just because certain medications are listed in the treatments doesn't mean you have to take them. They are there if needed. In fact, medications should be considered a last resort.

Mostly, the only medications mentioned in the diagnoses and treatments in this book are ones that have been listed here, but that does not mean they are the only options. Often there are many alternatives.

Self-medication can be dangerous, especially with prescription medication. If you have the option, always see a doctor before taking any medications.

Specific dosages are (mostly) only mentioned for those recommended in the first aid kit, and are only for healthy adults. Unless otherwise specified, they are for oral intake of instant-release drugs, as opposed to intravenous (IV), extended release, etc. If you plan to keep other medications in your first aid kit, and for pediatric doses or other complications (e.g., pregnancy, compromised immune systems), research must be done.

The specific use for each type of medication (e.g., when to use it, dosage) is given under the relevant sections in the Diagnoses and Treatments.

IMPORTANT: Recommendations often change when new research is done. If a medical professional is not available, it is best to consult the Physician's Desk Reference or Drugs.com for the latest information on which drugs to use and correct dosages. Dosages given in this book are mainly from www.drugs.com and are accurate at the time of publishing.

Related Chapters:

- First Aid Kit

ALTERNATIVE REMEDIES VS PHARMACEUTICALS

In general, pharmaceutical companies do not make money off of alternative remedies. This means that they do not spend money researching them; therefore, many alternative remedies have not been scientifically proven to be effective. That does not mean that they do not work. Actually, even proven pharmaceuticals may not solve certain problems. This is because we are all different, and therefore all medicines will affect people differently.

One of the biggest pros for using alternative remedies is that they usually have far fewer side effects than pharmaceuticals. This means that unless you are totally against the use of alternative medicines, there is usually no harm in trying them first. If it does not work, you can always try the pharmaceutical afterwards.

Scientifically proven medications are recommended in emergency situations

GENERAL SAFE USE INFORMATION FOR ALL MEDICATIONS

The following applies to all medications, unless specifically stated otherwise:

Check for Allergies

When unsure if a medication may cause an adverse reaction, test it first with a small dose in the manner that you would use it, e.g., oral, topical. Allergies may manifest as diarrhea, rash, respiratory problems, etc.

Expiration Dates

In most cases, using out-of-date medication will not have a negative effect. They probably just won't be as potent as they would be if used before the expiration date. Research has shown that many medicines are still acceptable for use 10 to 15 years after the expiration date (liquid forms, e.g., insulin, lose potency much more quickly). However, if you can update your medications, do so.

Follow Instructions and Warnings

Instruction and warning/caution labels on medications are there for a reason. Follow them strictly. If a doctor gives you advice about the medication (e.g., dosage), follow it.

For People Unable to Swallow Pills, e.g., Small Children

Pills can be crushed or emptied (if a capsule) into a cup of water and swallowed that way. It is best to use a smaller cup and then refill it to get all the residue particles. Flavoring can also be added if needed. Do not chew or make a liquid out of time-release capsules.

Know the Possible Side Effects

An apparent allergic reaction may not be an allergic reaction at all. It may be a known side effect that you just have to deal with while taking the medication. Also, if you know what the side effects may be, you can adjust your life around them. For example, if drowsiness is a side effect, don't drive.

Mark All Medications Well

If you take medications out of the packet (e.g., to save space), ensure you correctly label them along with dosage and any other pertinent information.

Medication May Mask Underlying Problem(s)

Treating symptoms without knowing the cause is dangerous and will usually result in slower healing and/or reoccurring problems. Treat the cause first, and then treat the symptoms.

Stick to the Recommended Dosages

Overmedication is extremely dangerous and will often result in a worse problem, perhaps even death. On the other hand, if you do not take enough (e.g., not completing a course of antibiotics), it may not completely eradicate the problem. The Physician's Desk Reference or Drugs.com can give you exact dosages for many ailments.

Store Medications Properly

Most medications keep best in cool, dry, dark places, and preferably in an opaque container as opposed to a clear one.

ANALGESICS, ANTI-INFLAMMATORY DRUGS, AND FEVER REDUCERS

General Cautions

- Check for allergies.
- Don't take if neurologically impaired.
- Use the least potent medicine to do the job.
- NSAIDs are non-steroidal anti-inflammatory drugs and are useful in injuries associated with swelling or other signs of inflammation.

Acetaminophen (Tylenol)

- Pain reliever and fever reducer in the case of infection, good for children.
- Adult dose: 1,000 mg every 6 to 8 hours.

Aspirin

- NSAID, pain-reliever, fever reducer in case of infection, and anti-inflammatory
- Cautions: Do not give aspirin to anyone under 20 years, unless specifically prescribed by a doctor.
- Side effects: Blood thinning, upset stomach
- Adult dose: 325 to 650 mg every 4 hours as needed, not to exceed 4 g/day.

Corticosteroids (Prednisone, Cortisone)

- Strong anti-inflammatory and analgesic
- Side effects: Acne, appetite loss, heartburn, increased sweating, insomnia, nausea, vomiting

- Adult dose: 5 to 60 mg per day in evenly divided doses 1 to 4 times/day.
- Also available as a topical cream

Cyclobenzaprine (Flexeril)

- Muscle relaxant and sedative
- Cautions: Do not use for persons under 15 years.
- Side effects: Constipation, dizziness, drowsiness
- Adult dose: 5 to 10 mg 3 times/day (start at 5 mg and increase if needed).

Hydrocodone (Vicodin)

- Strong pain relief, cough suppressant
- Side effects: Anxiety, blurred vision, constipation, dizziness, drowsiness, dry mouth, headache, nausea, ringing in ears, upset stomach, vomiting
- Adult dose: 5 mg every four to six hours.

Ibuprofen (Motrin, Advil)

- NSAID, pain reliever, fever reducer in the case of infection and anti-inflammatory
- Considered the weakest of the NSAIDs, but still very effective and with less severity of side effects; doses greater than 400 mg do not enhance effectiveness.
- Side effects: Blood thinning, stomach upset
- Adult dose: 200 to 400 mg every four to six hours as needed.

Lidocaine

- Topical gel

- Cautions: Do not cover more than 5 % total body surface area, and do not repeat use.
- Usually takes five to ten minutes to take effect.

Naproxen (Aleve)

- NSAID, pain reliever, fever reducer in the case of infection and anti-inflammatory
- Stronger than other NSAIDs but takes longer to work.
- Cautions: Take in fewer doses (as compared to other NSAIDs) with lots of water, not recommended for children under 15 years.
- Side effects: Blood thinning, upset stomach (more so than with aspirin)
- Adult dose: Naproxen sodium 220 mg every 8 hours as needed.

Oxycodone (Percodan)

- Extreme pain relief
- Cautions: High potential for addiction (opioid)
- Side effects: Constipation, diarrhea, dizziness, drowsiness, dry mouth, gas, headache, heartburn
- Adult dose: 5 to 15mg every four to six hours.

Alternative Analgesics, Anti-Inflammatory Drugs, and Fever Reducers

- **Ginger:** Ginger root tea may decrease inflammation and provide pain relief.
- **Herbal Teas:** Chamomile, mint, and rosemary teas (amongst others) are mild muscle relaxants.
- **Ice:** Apply topically to numb the skin.
- **Oatmeal:** Reduces healing-related itching. Add 1 to 2 cups of raw oats to a lukewarm bath as it is filling. Soak in

the bath for 15 to 20 minutes. Air dry so a thin coating remains on your skin. Repeat as needed.
- **Salicin:** Analgesic, anti-inflammatory, and fever reducer. Salicin is what aspirin is made from.
- **Tannin:** Tannin will soothe itching and promote healing. Wash the area with black or green tea. Use as a compress or poultice and apply topically.

Related Chapters

- Must Read > Medications Guide > Medicinal Plants

ANTIBIOTICS

There are many different types of antibiotics, and each of them is used at specific dosages for specific illnesses. Some can also be used as a preventative measure (prophylactics).

The antibiotics referred to in this book were specifically chosen because they are multi-purpose and/or commonly accessible in the world and/or can be substituted with veterinary equivalents. Only consider veterinary equivalents that have the antibiotic as the sole ingredient, and only use them as a very last resort.

Note the following:

- Alcohol consumption is not advised while taking antibiotics and for 3 days afterwards.
- Antibiotics help your body to fight bacteria, but they do not work with viral infections. Respiratory infections are more likely to be viral.
- Do not self-medicate/administer antibiotics unless there is no other option and you are 100% sure it is the right medication for the illness.
- Over-use of antibiotics can create resistant bacteria and may cause severe allergic reactions. Only use them as a last resort.
- There may be multiple antibiotics suggested in the treatments, but unless specifically directed, only use one.
- In *Diagnoses and Treatments*, dosage recommendations are only given for the first three of the antibiotics listed here because they are the ones recommended in the first aid kit.

Amoxicillin/Clavulanate (Augmentin)

- Cautions: Do not use if allergic to penicillin.
- Side effects: Diarrhea, gas, headache, nausea/vomiting, skin rash, or itching

Ciprofloxacin (Cipro)

- Cautions: Do not use for children under 8 or pregnant women.
- Side effects: Diarrhea, headache, nausea, trouble sleeping
- Veterinary substitute: Fish Flox

Doxycycline (Vibramycin)

- Cautions: Do not use for children under 8 or pregnant women.
- Side effects: Diarrhea, nausea, skin rash, vaginal itching or discharge
- Dose for general bacterial infection: 200 mg on the first day, given in two divided doses, then 100 mg/24 hours or 100 mg/12 hours for severe cases.

Amoxicillin (Amoxil)

- Cautions: Do not use if allergic to penicillin.
- Side effects: Diarrhea, nausea, stomach pain, swollen tongue
- Veterinary substitutes: Fish-Mox (250 mg), Fish-Mox Forte (500 mg)

Ampicillin (Pricipen)

- Cautions: Do not use if allergic to penicillin.
- Side effects: Headache, nausea, stomach pain, swollen tongue, thrush, vaginal itching or discharge
- Veterinary substitute: Fish-Cillin

Azithromycin (Zithromax)

- Side effects: Constipation, decreased sensation (e.g., hearing, smell, taste), diarrhea, dizziness, insomnia, nausea and vomiting, rash, stomach pain, tiredness

Cephalexin (Keflex)

- Cautions: Do not use if allergic to penicillin.
- Side effects: Diarrhea, dizziness, joint pain, nausea, tiredness, vaginal itchiness or discharge, vomiting
- Veterinary substitute: Fish-Flex (250 mg), Fish-Flex Forte (500 mg)

Cortisporin

- Otic Drops for external ear infections or ointment for topical use.

Erythromycin Ophthalmic Ointment (Romycin)

- Eye ointment for corneal abrasion, eye infections, and snow blindness
- Side effects: Blurred vision, eye stinging

Levofloxacin (Levaquin)

- Cautions: Stop use if tendon pain develops.
- Side effects: Dizziness, headache, gastrointestinal problems, insomnia, vaginal itching or discharge

Metronidazole (Flagyl)

- Cautions: Do not use for children under 8 or pregnant women.
- Side effects: Abdominal pain, cold symptoms (e.g., cough, sneezing), diarrhea, loss of balance, nausea and vomiting (especially if consuming alcohol), sore tongue, vaginal itching or discharge
- Veterinary substitute: Fish-Zole

Sulfamethoxazole / Trimethoprim (Bactrim)

- Cautions: Do not use for children under 8 or pregnant women, do not use if allergic to sulfa drugs.
- Side effects: Dizziness, insomnia, painful tongue, ringing in ears, vomiting
- Veterinary substitute: Bird Sulfa

Tetracycline (Sumycin)

- Cautions: Do not use for children under 8 or pregnant women.
- Side effects: Diarrhea, genital or rectal sores/swelling, nausea, oral sores, swollen tongue, trouble swallowing, vaginal itching or discharge, vomiting
- Veterinary substitute: Fish-Cycline

Related Chapters:

- First Aid Kit

ANTI-FUNGALS

Clotrimazole (Lotrimin)

- Clotrimazole is available as a cream, lozenge, lotion, powder, and vaginal suppository.
- Side effects: Foul-smelling discharge (vaginal cream), skin irritation, stomach pain, vomiting (lozenges)

Fluconazole (Diflucan)

- Cautions: Do not use if allergic to fluconazole. Do not use if you take cisapride, erythromycin, pimozide, or quinidine. Do not take more than one dose if pregnant.
- Side effects: Altered sense of taste, diarrhea, dizziness, headache, stomach pain

Ketoconazole (Nizoral)

- Cautions: Do not mix with other medications. Do not take if you have liver problems.
- Side effects: Breast swelling, decreased libido, dizziness, headache, nausea, stomach pain, skin rash, vomiting
- Veterinary substitute: Fish-Fungus

Miconazole (Monistat)

- Miconazole is available as a cream, lotion, powder, sprayable liquid, and suppository.
- Side effects: Foul-smelling discharge (vaginal cream), skin irritation, stomach pain

Alternative Antifungals

- Garlic
- Tannin

ANTIHISTAMINES

Diphenhydramine (Benadryl)

- Side effects: Depleted coordination, difficulty urinating, dizziness, dry mouth, drowsiness, headache
- Also available as a topical cream

Standard adult dosages of diphenhydramine:

- Allergic reaction: 25 mg to 50 mg (1 to 2 Benadryl capsules).
- Cough: 25 mg every 4 hours as needed, not to exceed 150 mg per day.
- Cold symptoms: 25 to 50 mg every 4 to 6 hours as needed, not to exceed 300 mg/24 hours.
- Extrapyramidal Reaction (drug-induced movement disorders): 25 to 50 mg every 6 to 8 hours.
- Insomnia: 25 to 50 mg at bedtime.
- Motion Sickness: 25 to 50 mg every 6 to 8 hours. Administer first dose 30 minutes before exposure to motion and repeat before meals and upon retiring for the duration of the journey.

Loratadine (Claritin)

- Loratadine is used for relief of allergic rhinitis (hay fever).
- Side effects: Dry mouth, fatigue, headache
- Adult dose: 10 mg once a day.

ANTISEPTICS

Povidone Iodine (Betadine)

- Cautions: Do not drink. Do not freeze or heat.
- Use 10% for topical use, dilute to 1% for wound cleaning.

Dakin's Solution

- For disinfecting skin wounds
- Cautions: Do not drink. Do not freeze or heat. Store at room temperature. Shelf life is only 3 to 4 days.
- Side effects: Skin irritation may occur.

To make Dakin's solution, add half a teaspoon (t) of baking soda to 4 cups of boiled/sterilized water.

Add bleach to reach desired strength.

- 3 teaspoons for wound cleaning
- 3 tablespoons for infected wounds
- 100 milliliters for bad infections

Alternative Antiseptics

- Alcohol: High-percentage drinking alcohols can be used if nothing else is available, preferably 50% alcohol by volume (ABV) or more, e.g., whisky or vodka. Do not use beer or wine. Lemon juice can also work for minor cuts.
- Garlic
- Honey: Especially good for burns

Using honey as an antiseptic:

- Liberally and completely cover affected area with honey so no air can get to it.
- Cover with cling wrap or waterproof dressings.
- Change dressing as needed, minimum of 3 times a day, do not wash off honey.
- Repeat until healed.
- Do not wash off the honey for up to 20 days (or earlier if healing is complete).

ANTIVIRAL DRUGS

Acyclovir (Zovirax)

- Side effects: Agitation, diarrhea, dizziness, hair loss, joint pain, lethargy, rash, upset stomach, vomiting

Famciclovir (Famvir)

- Side effects: Diarrhea, gastrointestinal problems, headache, lethargy, nausea, rash, skin irritation, vomiting

Oseltamivir (Tamiflu)

- Cautions: Tamiflu should not be used as a replacement for your annual flu immunization, only works if used within 2 days of symptoms appearing.
- Side effects: Diarrhea, dizziness, eye redness, headache, insomnia, nausea, nosebleed, respiratory problems, vomiting

Alternative Antivirals

- Garlic

HAEMOSTATICS

General Cautions: Only use if well-aimed direct pressure does not work.

Zeolite (QuikClot)

- Use as instructed on product package.

Styptic

- In pencil or powder form

Alternative Haemostatics

- Cayenne pepper powder
- Cinnamon powder

HIGH-ALTITUDE MEDICATIONS

Acetazolamide (Diamox)

- Acetazolamide is preferable as a preventative drug to be used before/during ascent.
- Cautions: Do not use if allergic to sulfa or penicillin, e.g., if a rash starts to develop a few days after ingestion.
- Side effects: Bitter taste of carbonated beverages, decreased blood clotting ability, depressed immune system, drowsiness, impotence, increased urine output, nausea, near-sightedness (myopia), tingling in hands and feet
- Adult dose for AMS (altitude sickness): 125 to 250 mg every 6 to 12 hours, maximum dose of 1 gram per day.

Dexamethasone (Decadron)

- Dexamethasone is better for treatment; take in conjunction for descent.
- Side effects: Dizziness, headache, insomnia, skin problems (acne, dryness, etc.)
- Adult dose for AMS: 0.75 to 9 mg per day in divided doses every 6 to 12 hours.

Alternative High-Altitude Remedies

- Coca leaves (tea or chewed) may help with altitude sickness.

MOTION SICKNESS, NAUSEA, AND VOMITING

Dimenhydrinate (Dramamine)

- Dimenhydrinate is an antihistamine.
- Side effects: Blurred vision (rare), drowsiness, dry mouth (rare), headache (rare), loss of coordination (rare)
- Adult dose: 50 to 100 mg every 4 to 6 hours, maximum of 400 mg in 24 hours. The first dose should be taken 30 to 60 minutes before starting activity.

Benadryl

Alternative Remedies for Motion Sickness, Nausea and Vomiting

- Ginger is well known for relief of motion sickness.

Related Chapters

- Must Read > Medications Guide > Antihistamines

MEDICINAL PLANTS

There are many medicinal plants, but this book only refers to a few of the more commonly found ones. Others are mentioned, but the main ones are garlic, ginger, and tannin.

Preparing Medicinal Plants

There are a few different methods mentioned in this book of preparing plants:

Direct consumption. Depending on the plant, you can eat it or just chew on it for the juice and spit the pulp out.

Poultice. Mash up the under-bark and shape it into a flat, pulpy mass. Add water if it is too dry. Apply it to the affected area, cover it (e.g., material, big leaf), and bind it in place.

Tea (infusion). Cut and crush the plant and put it in a cup. Pour boiling water over it, give it a stir, and then cover it. When cool enough, drink it. Depending on the plant, eat the ingredients after you finish drinking the tea.

If you cannot boil water, use cold water (half the amount) and leave it in the sun.

Salicin

Aspirin is made from salicin. It has analgesic and anti-inflammatory properties.

Find an aspen, poplar, or willow tree. There are various kinds of each, so the pictures may not match.

Chew on strips or make a tea from the green under-bark, as the outer bark is not effective.

A poultice can be used topically.

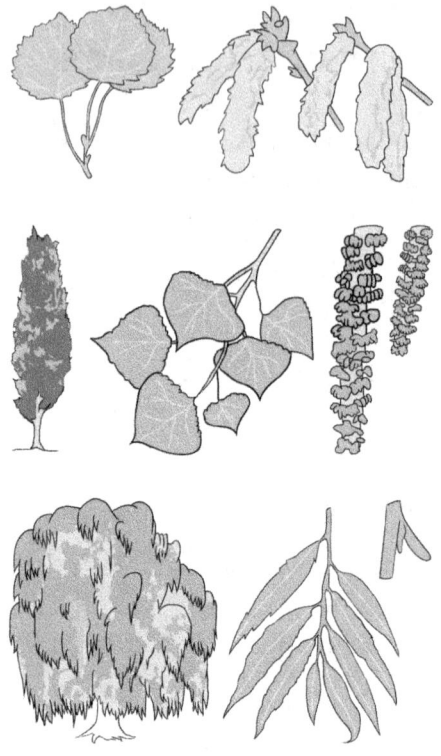

Tannin

Tannin has medicinal properties (e.g., it is an analgesic and can cure dysentery and promote healing) and can also be used to cure animal hides. Oak trees are best, but any tree will work.

- Boil tree bark (off the tree, not dead) for at least 12 hours and up to 3 days.
- Add more water as it evaporates.

Garlic, Ginger, Honey, and Lemon Tea

This tea gets a special mention because the ingredients are very common and it is a good natural remedy for when you have a cough or sore throat or feel a cold coming on. When you do not have all the ingredients, or even if you just have one, it can still help.

PART ONE: MUST-READ INFORMATION

Garlic. Eating two to three cloves of garlic a day (e.g., in cooking) is great for your immune system.

Cautions: May increase bleeding, so use with caution if you have stomach or digestion problems.

Garlic is known to help with the following:

- Bacterial infections and symptoms
- Blood pressure
- Blood sugar
- Fungal infections and symptoms
- Gastrointestinal infection and symptoms
- Hay fever
- Immune system
- Liver function
- Respiratory infections and symptoms
- Stress and fatigue
- Tick bites (prevention)

Ginger. Ginger has anti-inflammatory properties and is widely used as an anti-nausea remedy.

Cautions: Excess use may be harmful during pregnancy.

Ginger is known to help with the following:

- Gastrointestinal infection and symptoms
- Nausea/motion sickness/morning sickness
- Pain relief
- Respiratory infections and symptoms

Honey. Honey has antibacterial, anti-inflammatory, and antioxidant properties.

Honey (raw/unprocessed) is known to help with the following:

- Asthma
- Cough

- Diabetic foot ulcers
- Diarrhea
- Hay fever
- Lethargy
- Stomach ulcers
- Wound healing, including burns

Lemon. Lemon has anti-inflammatory and diuretic properties, i.e., increases urine output.

Lemon is known to help with the following:

- Cold and flu
- Digestion
- Kidney stones
- Pain
- Scurvy (vitamin C deficiency)
- Tinnitus (ringing in the ears)

Garlic, Ginger, Honey, and Lemon Tea. How much of each ingredient you put into the tea depends on how sick you are versus how much you can stand. Below is a sample recipe for a single cup. Eating the ingredients after your finish the tea is a good idea.

- 4 cloves of crushed garlic (peeled)
- Half a teaspoon of grated garlic
- A few tablespoons of lemon juice
- Raw honey to taste

MISCELLANEOUS

Hot Water and Rest

As a general rule, for any illness, unless instructed otherwise, rest and drink lots of water (preferably hot water) to flush your body of toxins and recharge your body.

If able, soak the affected part in hot water. An alternative for parts you cannot soak is to put something hot on them, e.g., brick, hot water bottle, rock.

Placebos

Placebos can be very powerful. Never tell a patient there is nothing that can be done. Doing something that has no proven benefit (and has no harmful effect) is better than doing nothing.

The Will to Live

No matter how dire a situation, you must keep up the will to survive. Don't just lie down to die. Keep going, do the best you can with what you have, find the humor in the situation, and keep up faith!

The moment you give up is the moment you have died.

IMMEDIATE FIRST AID

This section covers what to do medically in a life-threatening situation. Keep the patient alive until advanced medical care arrives.

Everyone should take a wilderness first responder course or, at the very least, a basic first aid course. Under no circumstances should this information replace a live first aid course conducted by a professional and qualified first aid instructor.

If possible, the first thing to do in all situations that require immediate first aid is to call emergency medical services. Know what the emergency services number is in whatever country you visit.

Something to think about:

The idea of first aid is to keep the patient alive until advanced medical care can be administered. In a survival situation, advanced care may not be available. Nursing a patient takes valuable time and resources.

If there is no possibility of advanced medical care, you may only be delaying an inevitable death and in the process taking away resources from other survivors.

Is it worth risking everybody? This is a choice you may have to make.

CRITICAL FIRST AID

This section will explain what to do when you first come across someone in need of first aid. It will allow you to determine urgent problems in the body's critical systems (i.e., circulatory, nervous, and respiratory).

Stop and fix problems as you find them. Some may be obvious, while others will need further investigation.

Although this is presented in a 'do this, then this' format, it is unlikely that you will be able to follow it smoothly in a medical emergency. You have to be flexible.

Whoever is the most qualified 'medic' on the scene is the one in charge; if someone comes along that is more qualified, that new person takes charge.

ASSESS THE SITUATION

When you come across any emergency situation, it is important to not rush in. To ensure the safety of you and everyone else, you must first assess the entire situation. Ensure the surroundings are safe for you, your rescue partners, the public, and then the patient(s)—in that order.

Next, try to determine what may have caused the situation and if there may be spinal damage to the patient. Knowing the cause will help you to determine likely injuries, predict further complications, and help you avoid getting injured by the same thing.

Finally, assess the number of patients, the need of additional rescuers, and what resources you have or need.

All this may seem overwhelming, but your brain is awesome. With some practice, and depending on the complexity of the situation, all this information can be gathered within seconds.

MENTAL STATUS: AVPU

Approach the victim and check his mental status using the acronym **AVPU**.

Gently shake the individual and ask loudly, "Hello, can you hear me? Are you okay?"

- **Alert:** Patient is awake.
- **Verbal:** Patient responds to verbal stimulus.
- **Pain:** Patient responds to pain stimulus.
- **Unresponsive:** Patient is unresponsive.

Anything below "Alert" may be the result of other critical system injuries or could also give rise to them. Assess with the secondary exam after critical first aid has been completed.

If you need to and are able, put on gloves and call for help.

Use the emergency roll to get the patient on his back and check his critical systems at the same time.

Emergency Roll

Vice-lock the patient's spine:

- Support the head and spinal column.
- Grasp the jaw and the back of the head, and squeeze the center line of the torso between your forearms.

Roll the patient onto her back.

For larger patients, use the heel of your foot to nudge the pelvis so that it rolls with the upper body.

PART ONE: MUST-READ INFORMATION

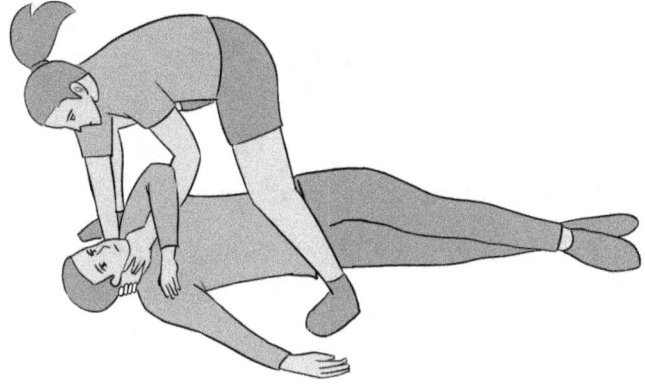

Move to the back of the patient and hover your closer hand over the mouth to check for breath.

At the same time, with your other hand, check the radial pulse which is located just below the wrist at the base of the thumb.

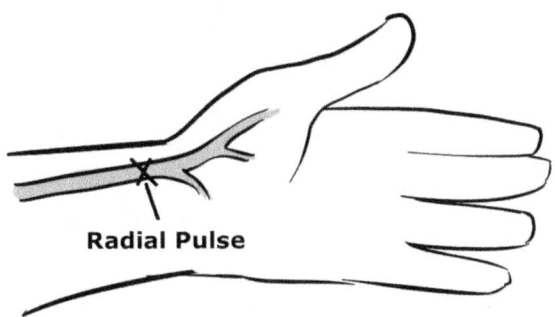

Note: Do not use your thumb to check for a pulse, as the thumb has a light pulse of its own.

Also check for and treat any severe bleeding.

Related Chapters

- Must Read > Secondary Exam
- Must Read > Critical First Aid > Circulation
- Must Read > Critical First Aid > Severe Bleeding

AIRWAY

Determine if air is moving in and out.

If the patient is breathing, air will be moving.

If you didn't notice it during the emergency role, put your ear close to the patient's face so that you are looking down his torso.

Place your hand on his abdomen and look, listen, and feel for signs of breathing.

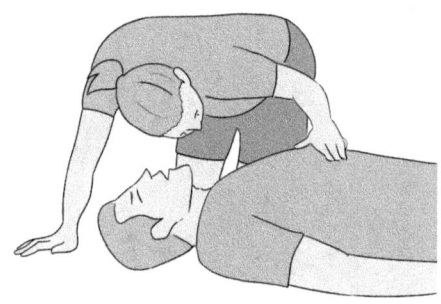

Chin Lift

If the airway is not open, use the chin lift.

Lift up the chin gently with one hand while pushing down on the forehead with the other to tilt the head back.

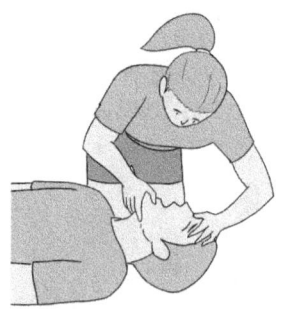

If you suspect a neck injury, open the airway using the chin lift without tilting the head back.

If the airway remains blocked, tilt the head slowly and gently until the airway is open.

With infants (under 1 year old) be careful not to tilt the head back too far, or it may block the breathing passage instead of opening it.

Finger Sweep

If the airway is still not open, check for a blockage.

If there is one, sweep your finger inside the patient's mouth to remove it. Be careful of his teeth.

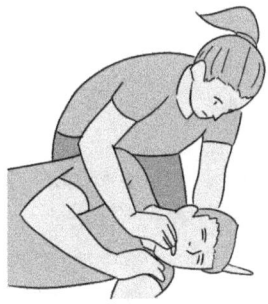

If there is any fluid (e.g., blood, water, vomit), use gravity to help drain it.

Support the patient's head and neck with one hand, and reach around to the center of his back with the other.

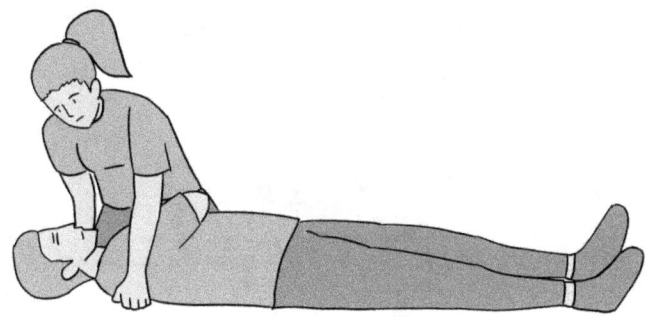

Roll the patient onto your thighs and clear the airway using the finger sweep if needed.

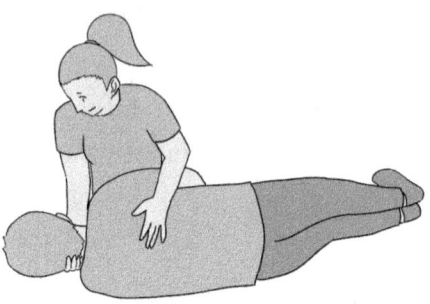

If the airway is being blocked due to swelling (e.g., trauma, burns, anaphylaxis), treat the cause (if possible).

Rescue Breathing

Next, give two rescue breaths.

Transmission of infection between rescuer and patient is extremely rare. As far as we know, HIV or AIDS has never been transmitted via rescue breathing. If you are worried, a barrier can be improvised by slitting a small hole in some sort of material, e.g., glove or plastic bag.

Pinch the person's nose shut using your thumb and forefinger. Your hand stays on the patient's forehead to maintain the head tilt. Your other hand also remains lifting up under his chin.

Inhale normally first (not deeply), and then form a tight seal between your mouth and the patient's mouth.

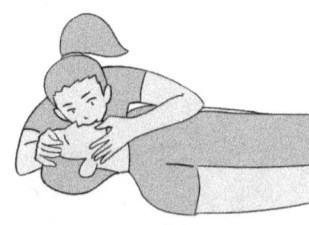

With your mouth tightly sealed on the patient's, slowly breathe into the patient's mouth for one second.

Provide two of these breaths.

If the patient's chest does not rise after the first breath, it means the air is not going in. Perform the head tilt again before attempting the second breath.

For small children:

- The breath for the child lasts for 1.5 seconds, and chest compressions are performed with these two rescue breaths.
- Be careful with your force of breath. Only use enough to make the chest rise.

For infants:

- Cover the nose and mouth with your mouth.
- The breath for the infant lasts for 1.5 seconds.
- Be careful with your force of breath. Only use enough to make the chest rise.

Abdominal Compressions

If the rescue breaths do not go in, it means there is still a blockage. Use abdominal compressions.

- Straddle the patient's legs.
- Place a fist or your palm heel between the breastbone and belly button.
- Thrust upwards up to five times to dislodge the obstruction.
- Attempt the rescue breaths again.
- Do five more abdominal compressions if needed, then two more rescue breaths.
- Repeat the five abdominal compressions and two rescue breaths until your breaths go in.

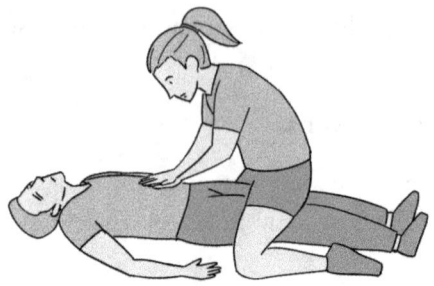

Related Chapters

- Must Read > Immediate First Aid > Critical First Aid > Circulation

BREATHING

If breathing is not adequate, treat the underlying cause (if possible).

PROP

- **Position:** Put the patient in a position of comfort
- **Reassurance:** Reassure the patient.
- **Oxygen:** Provide 100% oxygen if available.
- **Positive Pressure Ventilation** is artificial respiration by mechanical means. The non-mechanical equivalent is rescue breathing. Use one breath every 6 to 8 seconds, which is about 8 to 10 breaths a minute.

If there is no pulse, you will do CPR instead of just rescue breathing.

Related Chapters

- Must Read > Immediate First Aid > Critical First Aid > Airway
- Must Read > Immediate First Aid > Critical First Aid > Circulation

CIRCULATION

Pulse

If you didn't check pulse with an emergency roll, do so now. Lightly press the pads of your index and middle fingers on either the radial or carotid pulse. Do not use your thumb to check pulse since your thumb has a light pulse of its own.

The carotid pulse is located on the neck in the hollow between the windpipe and the large muscle.

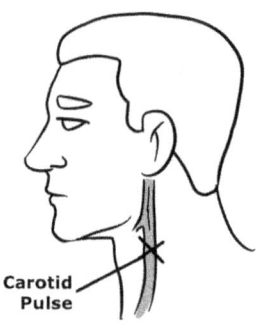

Cardiopulmonary Resuscitation

If there is no pulse, start CPR (cardiopulmonary resuscitation).

Don't waste time. If you are unsure about whether the heart is beating and you can't find a pulse within a few seconds, just start CPR.

CPR is the combination of chest compressions and rescue breathing.

During CPR, consider three things: airway, breathing, and circulation.

- Open the airway with the chin lift.

- Give two rescue breaths.
- Do 30 chest compressions at the rate of 100 compressions per minute.

Chest Compressions

Kneel at the patient's side near his chest.

Place the heel of your hand on his breastbone (sternum) between the nipples at the bottom of the ribcage, i.e., where there is a little notch.

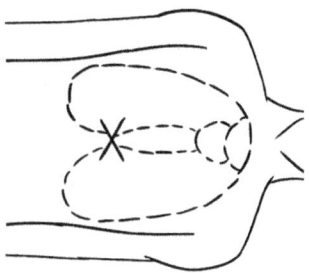

Place your other hand on top of the one that is in position. Lock your fingers together, pulling them up slightly so they are off the chest wall. Bring your shoulders directly over the person's sternum.

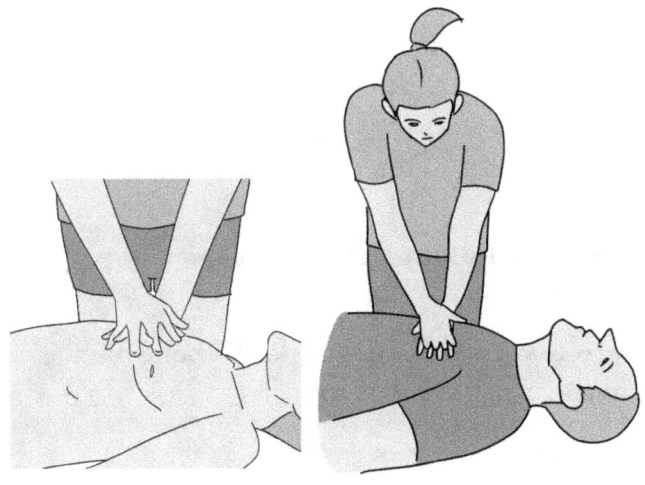

There are two parts to a chest compression:

- Compression (pushing down)
- Relaxation (releasing the chest back up)

Compression and relaxation should last for an equal length of time.

With your hands in position, press downward, keeping your arms straight.

Push down to about a third of the chest depth and then relax to let it return to the normal position.

Push hard and fast.

A cracking sound may be due to the ribs or cartilage cracking. Don't worry about it (for now); just keep doing the compressions.

Do 30 compressions for every two breaths at an overall rate of about 100 compressions per minute.

For an infant: Encircle your hands around the chest and use just your thumbs to do the compressions.

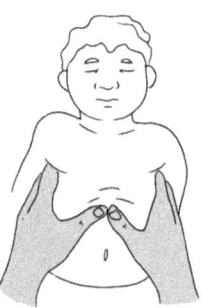

For children aged one to eight: Compress at about the nipple line.

If there are two rescuers: The person pumping the chest stops while the other gives rescue breaths.

If the victim starts to vomit: Turn the patient's head to the side and try to sweep out or wipe off the vomit, then continue with CPR.

When Not to do CPR

If advanced medical care is not readily available (e.g., more than 1 to 2 hours away), you need to make a decision whether to even start CPR or not.

To make a tough decision a little easier, you can follow these points as a standard. Do not start CPR if one or more of the following is found:

- The patient's core temperature is below 32 °C (90 °F).
- The patient has been underwater without air for more than 1 hour.
- The patient has an obvious lethal injury, e.g., massive hemorrhaging (severe bleeding must be stopped before giving compressions).

Also, any time that you do start CPR, you need to decide for how long you will continue. If advanced help is likely to arrive, then continuing until it arrives is reasonable.

If you are unsure whether help will arrive, then for how long should you continue? One hour? Two hours? These are decisions you have to make depending on the situation.

Perfusion

If CPR is not needed, check perfusion.

Perfusion is the flow of fluid (e.g., blood) through a certain area of the body.

Signs of inadequate perfusion include cold/clammy skin, altered mental status, slow capillary refill, and weak peripheral pulses (e.g., radial pulse).

If there is inadequate perfusion, treat the cause (if possible) and use PROP.

Testing Capillary Refill

Apply pressure to the skin and then wait to see how long it takes for blood to flow back into the site. A slow capillary refill indicates a slow return of blood and therefore decreased perfusion. A change in color from white to pink in less than 2 seconds is normal, while 3 or more seconds suggests that something might be wrong.

Good places to check capillary refill for general whole-body perfusion are the fingers and/or toes (especially at nail beds).

Related Chapters

- Must Read > Immediate First Aid > Critical First Aid > Airway
- Must Read > Immediate First Aid > Critical First Aid > Breathing

SEVERE BLEEDING

Well-Aimed Direct Pressure

Apply well-aimed direct pressure to the wound.

Elevate the wounded area above the heart if possible.

Wait ten minutes and then check if bleeding has stopped.

If it is spurting, stick your finger down on the wound and hold it there.

Pressure Point Constriction

If the patient continues to bleed after a period of well-aimed direct pressure, use pressure point constriction at an arterial pressure point between the injury and the heart. The closer to the bleeding site, the better.

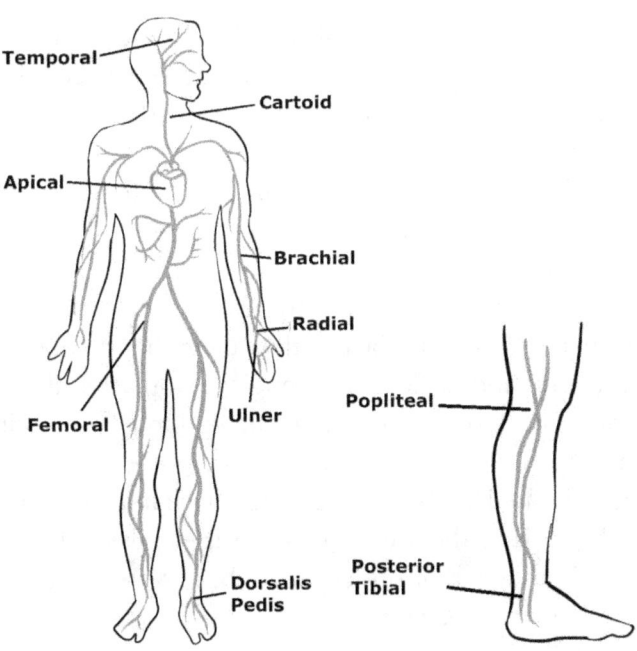

Do not perform pressure point constriction for more than 10 minutes as it can result in necrosis (death of body tissue). Be extra careful of the carotid artery, as occluding this artery hinders oxygen to the brain.

Tourniquet

If the patient is still bleeding, consider carefully whether to apply a tourniquet.

Note: This is a last resort. Only use a tourniquet if there is severe, uncontrolled bleeding that will cause loss of life and no other option is available and/or working.

Long-term use of a tourniquet may cause loss of the limb.

To apply an improvised tourniquet:

- Find a length of strong, pliable cloth, preferably no less than 5 cm (2 inches) wide, e.g., backpack strap, clothing, or long sock.
- Apply it on the limb, preferably with padding underneath, e.g., rolled-up clothing. It should be placed between the wound and the heart, approximately 5 to 10 cm (2 to 4 inches) from the wound.
- If possible, wrap it around the limb several times, keeping the material as flat as possible.
- Tie a simple overhand knot.
- Place a torsion device (e.g., a strong stick) on top of the knot, then secure it in place with two overhand knots.
- Twist the torsion device just enough to stop arterial (bright red) bleeding. Continued dark bleeding for a short while is normal in cases of amputation.
- Once tightened, secure the torsion device in place, e.g., loop the ends of the tourniquet over the ends of the stick and tie them together under the limb.
- Note what time you applied it.
- Do not cover it.

PART ONE: MUST-READ INFORMATION 87

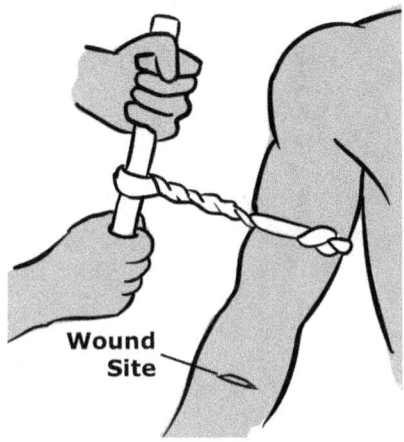

After 20 minutes of applying the tourniquet, ensure a pressure dressing is in place and that bleeding has stopped.

Very slowly loosen the tourniquet to restore circulation.

Leave the loosened tourniquet in position in case the bleeding resumes.

If transferring the patient to other caregivers (e.g., paramedics), write down the time at which you applied the tourniquet and the letters 'TK' on the patient's forehead.

Related Chapters

- Diagnosis and Treatments > Musculoskeletal System > Amputations

NERVOUS SYSTEM

The nervous system includes the brain and spine.

Checking mental status is the first things you should do after you assess the situation.

Spinal Injury

If you suspect a spinal injury or are unsure, do not move the patient unless absolutely necessary.

Protect and stabilize the spine.

Related Chapters

- Must Read > Immediate First Aid > Critical First Aid > Assess the Situation
- Must Read > Secondary Exam > Physical Exam > Spinal Assessment

ANAPHYLAXIS

Anaphylaxis is a life-threatening allergic reaction.

A history of mild allergic reaction does not mean you will never have a severe allergic reaction to the same thing. Often, the first time someone is exposed to an allergen, very little happens, but the second (or third, etc.) time there is a major reaction.

Symptoms usually show within minutes of exposure. The faster you treat them the better. Recurrent reactions can occur within 24 hours of the original episode. Treat these in the same way as the initial reaction.

Possible Causes of Anaphylaxis

- Drugs: More common ones are anesthetics, antibiotics such as penicillin, dyes injected during x-rays, heart and blood pressure medicines, and NSAIDs.
- Exercise: Often after eating
- Foods: Nuts, fruit, seafood, etc.
- Insect stings: Bees, wasps, etc.
- Latex: Rubber gloves, condoms, etc.

There are also many unknown causes.

Symptoms of Anaphylaxis

- Abdominal pain
- Decreased mental state
- Diarrhea
- Dizziness
- Hives
- Itching
- Nausea

- Respiratory problems
- Shock (rapid heart rate, low blood pressure, etc.)
- Skin redness
- Swelling of the mouth and face
- Paresthesia (tingling)
- Vomiting
- Weakness

Treatment for Anaphylaxis

- Diphenhydramine (e.g., Benadryl): 1 mg/kg of body weight, maximum of 50 mg, every 4 to 6 hours. Chewing the pill will make it work faster.
- Rescue breathing or CPR as needed

Administer epinephrine if:

- There is an obvious major reaction, e.g., difficulty breathing, unconsciousness.
- A reaction worsens over a few minutes.

Dosage of epinephrine: 0.01 ml/kg of body weight, maximum of 0.3 ml. Injections can be repeated every 5 minutes if needed.

- Administer diphenhydramine as soon as possible.
- Consider a corticosteroid (e.g., prednisone).

Dosage of prednisone: 1 mg/kg of body weight, maximum of 60 mg, once a day.

- Observe for at least 24 hours in case of secondary reaction.

If in doubt, administer the epinephrine.

Administering Epinephrine

The easiest way to do this is with a commercial injector, e.g., EpiPen. Patients that have a history of anaphylaxis will probably carry one with them. It is a good idea to have one in your first aid kit just in case, and they are usually allowed on planes.

These injectors have clear instructions written on them. Exact usage varies, but basically you remove the cap, hold it firmly in your fist, and press it firmly into the patient's thigh.

There is no need to stab the patient with it. That will just cause unnecessary bruising and pain.

Do not put your finger or thumb on the top of the device as you could accidentally inject yourself.

Epinephrine can also be given with a normal syringe.

HEART ATTACK

A heart attack (i.e., myocardial infarction, or MI) occurs when the heart is unable to get oxygen due to a blockage of blood flow. Aging people that do not keep in good health are most likely to suffer heart attacks.

Symptoms of Heart Attack

Symptoms vary from person to person and from case to case, i.e., the patient may not have the same symptoms as from a previous heart attack.

- Chest pain, tightness, or pressure
- Heartburn
- Indigestion
- Nausea
- Pain radiating to the jaw and right arm
- Shortness of breath
- Sweating
- Vomiting
- Weakness, dizziness, and light headedness

Treatment for Heart Attack

Seek advanced medical care as soon as symptoms of a heart attack are suspected. If in doubt, seek treatment.

- Aspirin: Chew in event of heart attack.
- Nitroglycerin: A patient with a history of heart attack may have this prescribed. Use as directed.
- Oxygen
- Rest

PRESSURE-IMMOBILIZATION TECHNIQUE

The pressure immobilization technique is used for only the most life-threatening venomous bites and stings. The idea is to slow the spread of venom into the circulatory system. This buys time until advanced medical care can be given.

The patient must be kept as still as possible, especially the site of the wound. Do not elevate the wound.

In general, only use the pressure-immobilization technique for:

- Australian snakes, all species
- Blue-ringed octopus
- Conus
- Funnel-web spiders

Applying the Pressure-Immobilization Technique

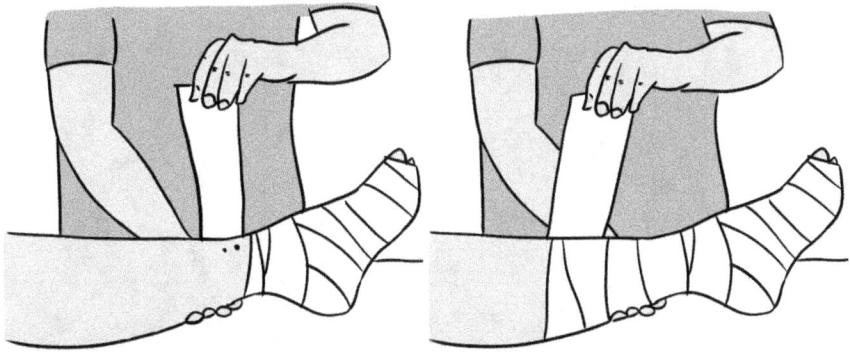

Ideally, use an elastic roller bandage.

- Bandage upwards from the lower portion of the bitten or stung limb, and continue up as high as possible.
- Each wrap should overlap the last.
- Ensure the bandage does not impair perfusion.
- Mark the location of the bite on the bandage.

- Immobilize the limb.
- Check perfusion frequently as continued swelling may impair it.

Note: Do not bandage bites/stings to the head or torso. Keep the patient still, and seek medical care ASAP.

Related Chapters

- Diagnosis and Treatments > Musculoskeletal System > Immobilization

SUCKING CHEST WOUND

Assume any penetrating wound to the chest is a sucking chest wound.

Symptoms of a Sucking Chest Wound

- Bloody froth
- Patient gasping for breath
- Sucking sound

Treatment for a Sucking Chest Wound

- Seal the wound with airtight material, taping only three sides so air can escape but not enter.
- If no airtight material is available, use your hand.
- Monitor the patient's breathing and check the dressing regularly.
- You can aid breathing by lifting the untaped side of the dressing as the patient exhales.

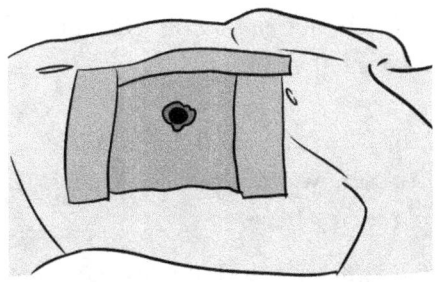

MASS CASUALTY CRITICAL ASSESSMENT

In the case of disaster, there is a good chance of multiple casualties.

A mass casualty incident is defined as any event where your medical resources are inadequate for the number and severity of injuries incurred.

If you choose to help, your goal is to do the greatest amount of good for the greatest number of people while keeping yourself and other rescuers safe.

Assess the situation as you normally would.

Quickly assess and 'tag' each patient. You can tag with numbers or colors. There is no international standard, but the following method is well recognized (U.S. standard):

- **1 or Red:** Highest priority. Probable loss of life or limb if immediate medical care is not given.
- **2 or Yellow:** Needs medical care but can wait 2 to 4 hours. Patient may enter red category over time.
- **3 or Green:** Minor injuries. Referred to as the "walking wounded." Can help with other patients.
- **4 or Black:** No chance of saving. Do not initiate CPR unless the cause is lightning.

Depending on your situation and/or resources, tags that would otherwise be red or yellow may become black. Lack of advanced medical care is a big factor here.

Fix critical problems quickly if possible, but do not spend very much time on any one patient, preferably less than 30 seconds.

Tell each patient who you are and that you are there to help. Stay calm and reassure them.

Mass Casualty Primary Assessment Flow Chart

Open airway if necessary:

- If victim begins breathing once the airway is restored, tag red.
- If patient's respirations are too slow or too fast, tag red.
- If airway is open but they are not breathing, tag black.

If breathing is normal, check pulse and perfusion:

- If there is no pulse or capillary refill takes longer than 2 seconds, tag red.

If pulse is present and capillary refill is normal, move to mental status:

- If patient is unconscious or disorientated, tag red (explosions may cause temporary hearing loss, which is different from disorientation).
- If they can follow commands but are unable to get up, tag yellow.
- If they follow commands and can get up, tag green.

While doing the above, consider the following:

- Elevate legs if there are signs of shock.
- If there is any doubt as to the category, always tag as the highest priority triage level, e.g., if you are not sure between yellow and red, tag red.
- Once you have identified someone as level 1/red, tag them and move immediately to the next patient unless you have major bleeding to stop.
- Only administer CPR if you have sufficient resources.
- Protect the spine only if resources are available.

- Stop severe bleeding (use a bystander if available). If bleeding doesn't stop, tag red.

Once critical assessment and tagging have been completed, move patients in order of priority to a safe area for further treatment and secondary exams.

Related Chapters

- Must Read > Immediate First Aid > Critical First Aid > Assess the Situation
- Must Read > Secondary Exam

SECONDARY EXAM

Once all the critical issues have been addressed, you can move onto the secondary exam.

Unlike critical first aid where you treat the problems as you find them, with the secondary exam you complete the full assessment and then treat patients in order of priority.

The assessment comprises three stages: physical exam, SAMPLE history, and vital signs. The order in which you do these depends on the situation.

While conducting your exam, let the patient know what you are doing and record your findings.

RECORDING YOUR FINDINGS

Use the acronym **SOAAP** to record your findings.

- **Subjective information:** History, scene, story, and symptoms
- **Objective information:** Exam findings, vital signs
- **Assessment:** All the problems you found
- **Anticipated Problems:** Any problems that may arise
- **Plan:** What you are going to do

Write the patient's personal details at the top, including name, age, sex, birth date, weight, phone number, etc.

There are many SOAAP (SOAP) note templates you can download from the internet, but a pencil and paper is really all you need.

PHYSICAL EXAM

To conduct a physical exam, first examine the areas for which the patient has a specific complaint. Compare any outer physical complaints to the patient's non-injured side.

Check range of motion, circulation, motor skills, sensation, etc. Be very careful about forcing something to move or performing an action that is beyond the patient's capability.

Depending on the circumstances, a full-body physical exam may be needed to discover problems of which the patient may not be aware.

Do this in a systematic manner, from head to toe. Use only as much physical pressure as is necessary to discover injury or lack thereof. Check the whole body for obvious signs of injury, e.g., bumps, bruises, or bleeding.

A stethoscope, pen light, gloves, and tongue depressor will be useful.

Head

- Bumps, bruises, bleeding from orifices, etc.

Eyes

- Redness, whether the pupils respond equally to light

Mouth (inside and outside)

- Redness, sores, dental issues

Neck

- All around neck and back of the head, neck bones (vertebrae)

Chest

- Use a stethoscope if available and check lungs for abnormal sounds, e.g., wheezing, gurgles, crackles.

Heart

- Rhythm of heartbeat, e.g., fast, slow regular, or irregular

Ribs

- Possible fracture

Armpits

- Injury, parasites (lice, ticks, etc.), tenderness

Breast

- Move your fingers in a circular motion over the breast tissue, starting where the arm connects to the shoulder and ending at the nipple.

Abdomen

- Press on the abdomen with your open hand checking for pain, tenderness, swelling, abnormal masses, etc.
- Listen for bowel sounds and note if there is too much or

too little.
- Check percussion by placing your open hand on the different quadrants of the abdomen and tapping on your middle finger. It should sound hollow.

Liver and Spleen

- Press down on the patient's right side below the rib cage to determine if the liver is enlarged (you won't feel it if it isn't).
- An enlarged spleen will appear as a mass on the left side under the bottom of the rib cage.

Spine

- Check along the patient's spine for evidence of pain or injury. Never press directly on the vertebrae.

Kidneys

- Pound lightly with a closed hand on each side of the back below the last rib. An injury or infection of the kidneys will result in pain.

Extremities

- Check each extremity by feeling the muscle groups for pain or decreased range of motion.
- Check perfusion.
- Check for sensation by lightly tapping with sharp and dull sensations on all four extremities (hands and feet), e.g., by using a safety pin.

General Strength

- Place your hands on the patient's thighs and ask them to lift up.
- Ask the patient to grasp your fingers with each hand, and then try to pull your hand away; if you can't, that's good.
- Strength should be about equal on both sides of the body.

Spinal Assessment

If you suspect a spinal injury, e.g., a large fall, and the situation allows, you can perform a spinal test. In a survival situation, this can help you determine whether you need to stabilize the person's spine before moving them.

To rule out a spinal injury, the patient should meet the following criteria:

- **Reliable:** Cooperative, sober, alert, and free of distracting injuries
- **No spinal pain**
- **No numbness or tingling**
- **No spinal tenderness:** Using slight pressure, press down the patient's back to the sides of the vertebrae; never press directly on the vertebrae.
- **Normal motor/sensory function** in all four extremities, done during the extremities test in the physical exam. This does not apply if the extremity has a specific injury that would affect the outcome, e.g., broken wrist.

Spinal Stabilization

If the spinal test cannot be passed, stabilize the spine.

Keep the neck and back as stable as possible.

Note: A collar alone does not stabilize the spine.

Consider stabilizing the patient's spine while he/she is on his/her side, especially if the patient is already like that or you have to leave him/her.

Before you stabilize the spine, you may have to bring the body back into its correct anatomical position, i.e., standing straight with legs together and arms down the sides but with the patient lying down, preferably on his/her back.

- Be very careful.
- Move only one body part at a time.
- Undo kinks.
- Straighten joints.
- Position arms and legs close to the body.
- Stop if increased pain or resistance is met.

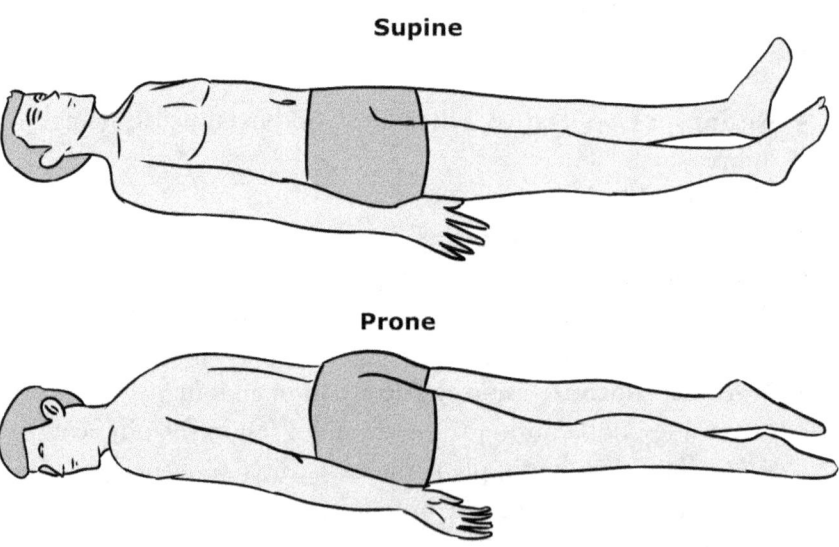

If moving the patient, it is preferably to secure him/her to a rigid litter.

PART ONE: MUST-READ INFORMATION

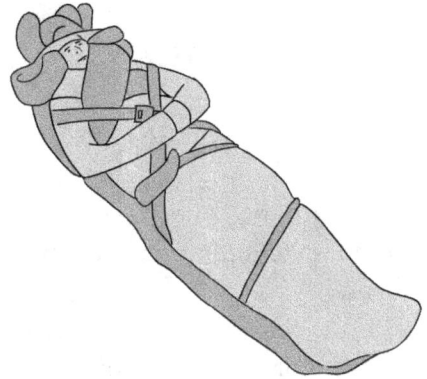

A rolled-up blanket, sleeping mat, or stuff-sack filled with sand (or similar) are just a few ways you can improvise head stabilization.

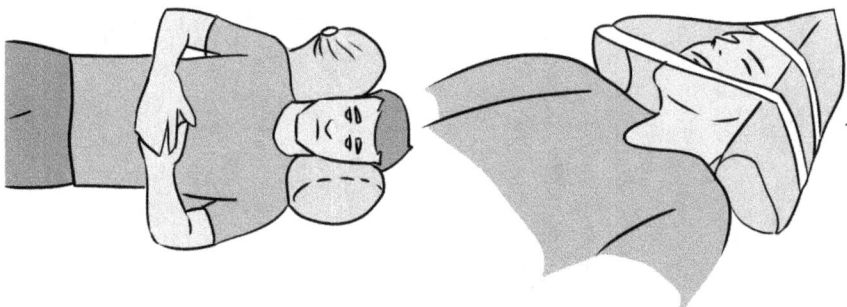

Related Chapters

- Must Read > Moving a Patient > Improvised Litters > Rigid Litters
- Must Read > Immediate First Aid > Critical First Aid > Circulation

HISTORY

Talk to the patient. Use the acronym **SAMPLE:**

- **Symptoms:** What are the patient's symptoms?
- **Allergies:** Does the patient have any known allergies (including medication)?
- **Medications:** Is the patient on any medication?
- **Past History:** Is the problem reoccurring, or does the patient or their family have a history of a suspected ailment?
- **Last Oral Intake and Output:** A history of the most recent things that went into and out of the person's body.
- **Events:** A detailed description of the events that led up to the problem.

VITAL SIGNS

Pulse

- Count the pulse for 15 seconds and multiply it by 4.
- Normal rate is 60 to 100 beats per minute.

Respirations

- Evaluate for an entire minute.
- Normal rate of breaths per minute (BPM) for an adult at rest is 12 to 18 breaths per minute. Over 20 BPM is a sign of distress.
- In children, the younger the child, the faster their respiratory rate—e.g., an infant may have 30 to 60 breaths per minute whereas a school-aged child (6 to 12 years) may have 18 to 30.
- Note any unusual noises, e.g., wheezing or gurgling.

Blood Pressure

- Check blood pressure if the equipment is available.
- Blood pressure measures the amount of work the heart has to do to pump blood throughout the body.
- A reading of less than 140/90 at rest is normal. It may be high after extreme physical exertion but should go back down after a short while.
- High blood pressure may be a medical condition, and low blood pressure may indicate hemorrhage or shock.

Skin

- Check color (red, pale), temperature (hot, cold), and moisture (clammy, dry, moist, etc.).

Body Temperature

- A normal temperature ranges between 36.1 °C (97 °F) and 37.2 °C (99 °F).
- A temperature above 38 °C (100.4 °F) or below 35 °C (95 °F) indicates that there is something wrong. Hyper- or hypothermia may be an issue.

Mental Status

Gauge with AVPU.

If there is a problem with the patient's mental status, use the acronym **STOPEATS** to discover the cause:

- **Sugar:** Hypo or hyperglycemia
- **Temperature:** Hypo or hyperthermia
- **Oxygen:** Abnormal levels of oxygen
- **Pressure:** Increasing intracranial pressure (ICP)
- **Electricity:** Trauma from electric shock or problems in the brain
- **Altitude:** High altitudes can result in various altitude-related illnesses, and very low altitudes (i.e., under water) can result in various diving-related illnesses.
- **Toxins:** Drugs, alcohol, poisons, etc.
- **Salts:** Low sodium or potassium levels

Related Chapters

- Must Read > Immediate First Aid > Critical First Aid >

Circulation
- Diagnosis and Treatments > Environmentally Induced
- Must Read > Immediate First Aid > Critical First Aid > Mental Status: AVPU
- Diagnosis and Treatments > Circulatory System
- Diagnosis and Treatments > Head > Brain > Increasing Intracranial Pressure
- Diagnosis and Treatments > Environmentally Induced > Altitude Induced
- Diagnosis and Treatments > Environmentally Induced > Cold and/or Water Induced > Diving Induced

OPEN WOUNDS, SKIN INFECTIONS, AND SEPSIS

Proper wound care is very important in the treatment of many things. Wounds that are not cared for properly can lead to cellulitis (bacterial skin infection), which can then lead to sepsis, a life-threatening condition.

OPEN WOUNDS

An open wound is wound that breaks the skin, e.g., cuts, scrapes, abrasions, and punctures.

Treatment for Open Wounds

- Control bleeding with well-aimed direct pressure.
- Clean.
- Cover with a sterile dressing.
- Immobilize high-risk wounds if possible.
- Change the bandage and clean the wound regularly.
- Monitor for infection and treat as needed.

Open Wound Care

Any open wound must be cleaned in order to minimize the chances of infection.

Use a combination of the following measures depending on the situation:

- Remove all foreign materials as best as you can.
- Wash the wound and the surrounding skin with soap and water. Lightly scrub.
- Irrigate the wound with at least 100 ml (ideally 1000 ml) of the cleanest water available, and make a final wash with water of drinking quality. Hot water (not scalding) is best.
- If there is foreign material that cannot be irrigated or there isn't enough water, rinse the wound out with antiseptic, e.g., Betadine.
- Cover the wound with a sterile dressing. Any adhesive should not actually touch the wound.
- If needed and possible, close the wound with sutures, staples, etc.

- Change dressings at least twice a day. If bandage is saturated, additional changes may be required.
- Clean the wound with clean drinking water (preferably with no chemicals) every time you change the dressing.
- If you see bleeding while changing the dressing, apply pressure until it stops.

If in the wilderness and/or a survival situation, it is best not to close a wound. The scar will be bigger, but there will be less chance of infection.

Wet-to-Dry Dressing

A wet-to-dry dressing may not be needed for minor wounds, but it can be very beneficial for larger ones.

- Soak a bandage in sterilized (boiled) water and wring the water out.
- Apply it directly onto the wound.
- On top of that, place a dry bandage.
- Secure it in place.

Debridement

During the healing process, you may see blackish material on the edge of the wound, and this must be removed. You can scrub it out, or you may need to trim it off.

IMPALING OBJECTS

An impaling object is an item that punctures the skin and is still inside and protruding from the patient, e.g., a knife.

Treatment for Impaling Objects

- Remove all impaling objects unless doing so would cause further harm.
- Exceptions include impaling objects in the globe of the eye or those whose removal would result in severe pain or bleeding.
- After removal, clean and treat as an open wound.

Related Chapter

- Must Read > Open Wounds, Skin Infections, and Sepsis > Open Wounds

SKIN INFECTION AND SEPSIS

Any wound is susceptible to infection, especially if not cared for properly. If an infected wound is not treated, it can lead to sepsis and, consequently, death.

Symptoms of Local Skin Infection

These symptoms are present at the site of the infection:

- Bad odor
- Discomfort/pain
- Heat on touch
- Pus and/or a cloudy fluid
- Redness
- Swelling
- Tenderness

Treatment for a Local Skin Infection

- Rest and elevate the infected limb.
- Drain the puss, incise if needed.
- Irrigate.
- Warm water soaks can be soothing.
- Consider immobilization of the limb.

The body can sometimes resolve the infection on its own, i.e., without pharmaceuticals. The chances of this are better if the wound is cleaned well.

- Antibiotic: Amoxicillin/clavulanate 500 mg every 12 hours for 7 days or for 3 days following resolution of acute inflammation, or 875 mg every 12 hours for 7 days or until 3 days following resolution for severe cases.
- Antibiotic: Ciprofloxacin 500 mg every 12 hours for 7 days

or until 3 days following resolution, or 750 mg every 12 hours for 7 days or until 3 days following resolution for serious cases.
- Antibiotics, other: Amoxicillin, ampicillin, cephalexin, levofloxacin, metronidazole
- Plantain leaves: Poultice
- Tannin: Compresses or direct application
- Honey: Topical application

Symptoms of Systemic Infection (Sepsis)

- Blistering
- Fatigue
- Fever and chills
- Malaise (general sick feeling)
- Muscle ache
- Pain
- Red streak

Treatment for Systemic Infection (Sepsis)

- Same treatment as local skin infection
- Consider surgical draining (advanced medical care will be needed).
- Antibiotic: Ampicillin

Related Chapters

- Diagnosis and Treatments > Integumentary System > Abscesses

MOVING A PATIENT

Moving a patient should only be done if absolutely necessary, especially if they are not in a stable condition. When moving, your aim is to cause the least amount of trauma to the patient and yourself.

If there is a suspected spinal injury, it is always better to move the patient along the long axis of the body.

DRAGS

Drags are best used over a short distance and fairly smooth terrain. They are useful if the situation is time sensitive and/or the patient is too heavy to carry. Be careful when walking backwards.

Basic Drag

Pull the patient by his/her clothes or from under his/her arms. The patient's head rests on your forearms.

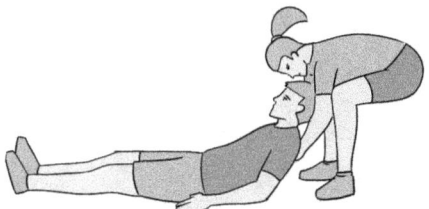

Blanket Drag

Roll the patient onto a blanket or something similar (raincoat, tent, etc.). Pull the blanket with the patient on it to safety.

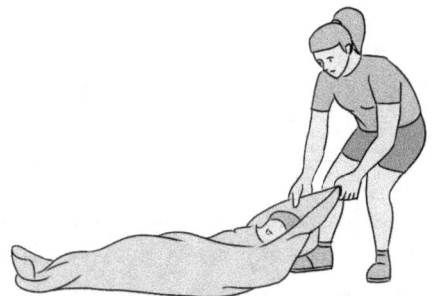

CARRIES

To prevent injury to yourself when lifting a patient (or any heavy object), keep your back straight and lift with your legs.

Avoid twisting and keep the weight close to your body.

Move in smooth motions, i.e., avoid jerking.

Backpack Carry

Essentially, the patient is placed into a backpack, and you put the patient on your back like you would a backpack. Cut leg holes in the base of the pack if needed.

Chair Carry

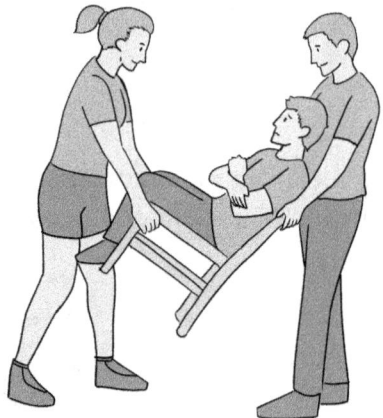

At least two rescuers are needed for a chair carry. The patient is carried while sitting in a chair. One rescuer lifts the back of the chair while the other lifts the front legs.

Fireman's Carry

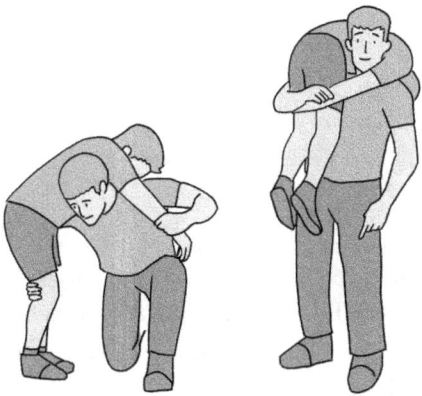

This can be difficult if the patient is larger than you.

Crouch down and grab the patient's right wrist with your left hand and position it over your shoulder.

Wrap your arm around the patient's legs (or between them) to grab around the patients' right thigh.

Stand up (using leg muscles) and adjust the patient's weight to a balanced and comfortable position.

Four-Hand Seat

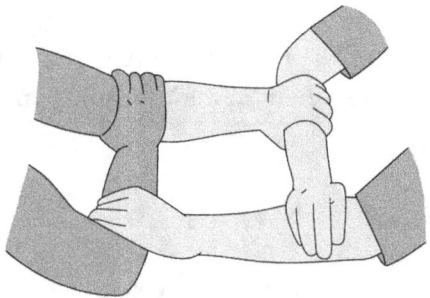

Two rescuers use their arms to create a 'seat' on which the patient can sit and be carried to safety. The patient must be able to support himself/herself by extending their arms around the rescuers' backs.

Each rescuer holds his/her own left forearm with the right hand, palm facing down.

The two rescuers then use their free hands to grab each other's respective forearms in order to make a square for the patient to sit on.

Improvised Harness Carry

The improvised harness carry is a secure way to carry a patient on your back. Place padding between the harness and the patient's body for comfort, especially around the shoulder straps.

Find some type of rope about 50 cm (20 in) long. The wider the better (within reason). Thick webbing is ideal.

Make a bight (loop) in the center of the webbing. Put this loop through the patient's legs, from back to front. The ends wrap behind each leg respectively and then pass through the loop at the front.

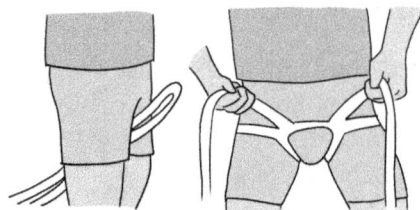

Kneel down in front of the patient with your back towards him/her. Bring the two ends over your shoulders and then back through the patient's legs.

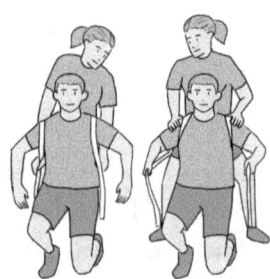

Loop to the outside of the patient's legs and tie the ends together just below your chest so it is tight but comfortable.

Pass the ends through their respective shoulder straps and then tie them off.

Papoose Sling

The papoose sling is useful for carrying infants and small children.

Tie a rectangular piece of material around your waist and neck to form a pouch at either your front or back.

Place the child inside.

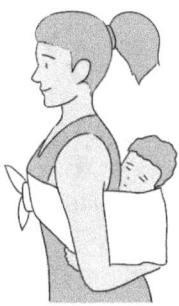

Piggyback

The patient climbs onto your back and holds on. If the patient is unconscious, you can grab the patient's arms and cross them around your chest. While keeping a straight back, lean forward slightly to help lift the patient off the ground.

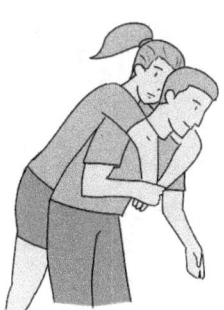

Supported Piggyback

A length of rope (approximately 5 m in length) or similar material can be used to support a patient that you piggyback. A wider material will add comfort as well as padding.

Place the center of the rope behind the patient and bring the ends forward under each armpit. The ends come over your shoulders and then wrap around the patient's thighs before being secured around your waist.

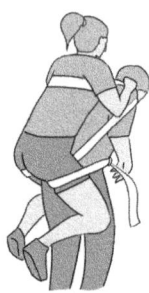

Two-Person Carry

One rescuer hugs the patient from behind at his/her chest.

The second rescuer positions in front of the patient and faces away from him/her, lifting the patient's legs.

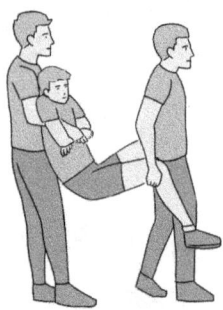

Wheelbarrow Carry

The wheelbarrow carry requires three rescuers. It is good for long distances.

Two rescuers stand next to each other, facing the direction of travel. The patient places his/her arms over these two rescuers' shoulders.

A third rescuer positions in front of the patient, also facing the direction of travel, and carries the patient's legs over his/her shoulders.

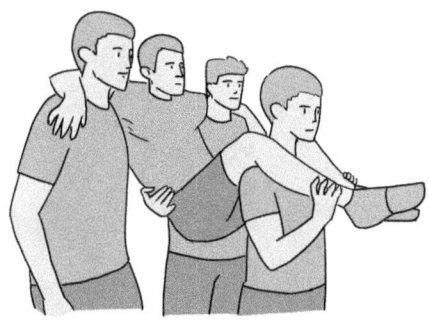

IMPROVISED LITTERS

There are two basic types of litters, non-rigid and rigid.

Non-rigid litters are faster to improvise but are not good for those with potentially critical injuries.

The improvised rigid litter is used when all other methods of transporting the patient are unsuitable.

It is never good practice to move a patient with a suspected spinal injury in any improvised litter, but if there is no way around it, a rigid litter is preferable.

Should there be a doubt about what to use, use a rigid litter.

Ensure spinal stabilization.

When moving the patient, move in small increments, preferably using axial movement as opposed to sideways movement.

The person at the head calls the movement.

Extra care must be taken when making a stretcher for a person with a possible spinal injury. Pad it well. The patient must be very well secured, i.e., unable to slide. You can achieve this by crossing straps and padding any gaps.

Related Chapters

- Must Read > Secondary Exam

PATIENT PACKING

When transporting patients in an improvised litter:

- Elevate the injured limb.
- Elevate the head slightly.
- Keep legs elevated if in shock.
- Lay unconscious patients on their sides.
- Give them something to hold.

When securing the patient, you can use padding (blankets, sleeping bags, clothes, etc.) to increase comfort, stability, and insulation. When doing so:

- Allow them to see what is happening around them.
- Construct a diaper if needed.
- Ensure the litter is easily moved.
- Ensure the patient is still accessible for assessment.
- Place some padding under the knees to prevent full extension.
- Protect the patient from the environment, e.g., falling debris.

NON-RIGID LITTERS

Many different non-rigid litters can be made depending on what you have available, e.g.:

- Branches and heavy duty parkas.
- Paddles with life jackets.
- Poles and packs.
- Poles with rope.

Blanket Litter

The items needed are two fairly straight pole-like objects, e.g., branches, and a large blanket or similar, e.g., tent, tarp.

Wrap the blanket around the poles as many times as possible. The more times you wrap it, the more secure it will be. The patient's weight holds it all together.

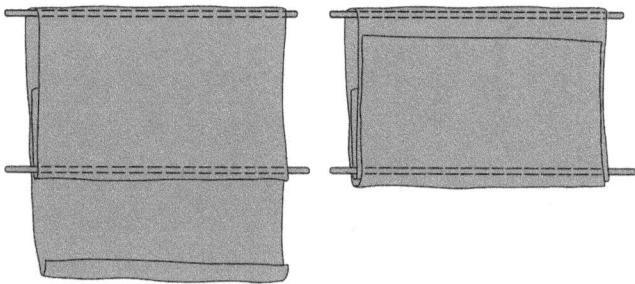

Rope Litter

An entire litter can be made of rope if needed.

Lay the rope on the ground in a zigzag-type formation, forming approximately 8 loops on the left and 8 loops on the right. The total length should be about the same size as the finished litter.

PART ONE: MUST-READ INFORMATION

Ensure you have enough rope left over on either end to tie off each loop. Make sure the loops won't slip through these tied-off knots. A clove hitch works well.

Thread the leftover rope through the ends of the loops. This ensures the knots won't slip off the bends. Tie the ends off.

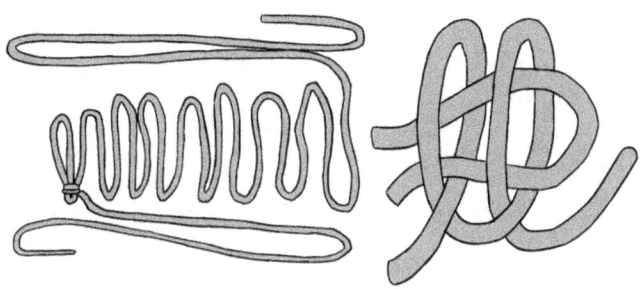

Improvements can be made by using poles and adding lots of padding.

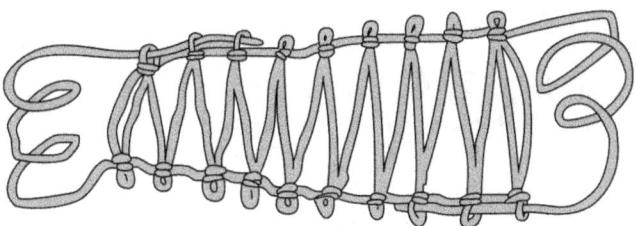

RIGID LITTERS

Kayak Litter

A kayak can create a great rigid litter but requires destroying the kayak if it does not have an open deck.

Remove the seat, flotation materials, and the upper deck if needed.

Mummy Litter

This type of litter is sturdier than most improvised litters, and adding more insulation (e.g., a sleeping bag) can help if the patient is suffering from hypothermia or a similar condition.

The downside is that the patient is severely restricted and enclosed, which may have a claustrophobic effect.

The following equipment is needed:

- Padding (sleeping pads, clothing, etc.)
- Poles (skis, paddles, branches, etc.)
- Rope
- Tarp (blanket, etc.)

Lay the rope out in U-shaped loops that taper off at the ends.

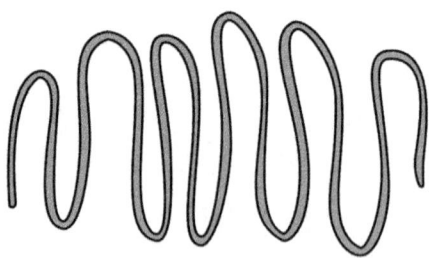

Tie a loop at the front end of the rope.

Put the tarp on top of the rope.

Next, place the pads down, then lay the poles out as the patient would lie.

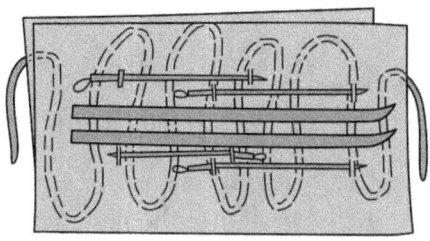

Put lots of padding on top of the poles, and then the patient goes on top of the pads.

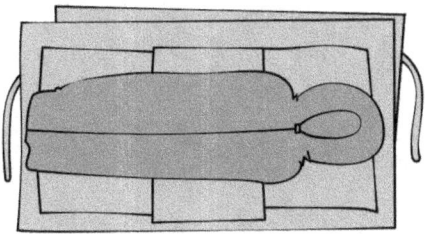

Close the daisy chain by bringing one loop through the pre-tied loop and then continuing to 'thread' these loops together to enclose the patient.

Once you reach the patient's armpits, bring a loop over each shoulder and tie it off.

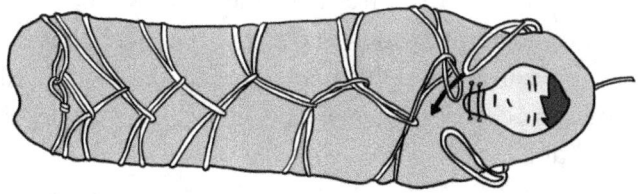

Pack Short-Board

This method will work with either an external or internal framed backpack.

Turn the pack 'face' down. The patient lies on the pack with his/her head on the padded hip belt. Secure the patient to the pack.

The hip belt can be used to strap down the patient's head. Put lots of padding between the hip belt and the patient's head if possible.

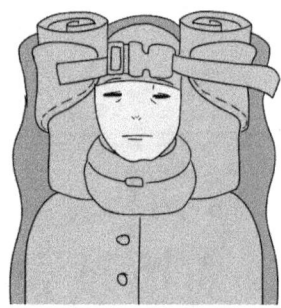

Carrying a Litter

The more people you have to carry the litter the better.

Ideally, you will have four to six people actually carrying the litter, as well as two people clearing the path.

Extra people are useful to rotate the carriers. It can be done without stopping (carefully) with the fresh people coming in from the back. Everyone then moves up, which allows the two people at the front to have a rest. These two people then move to the back. This can be done continuously so that everyone gets a periodic rest from carrying the litter.

The patient is usually carried feet first in the direction of travel. One exception might be when going uphill, in which case the head should be higher.

Frequently check vital signs.

For high-angle elevation, i.e., if ropes are needed, ensure the patient is well secured to the litter.

Improvised Sled/Sledge/Toboggan

Constructing an improvised sled-type vehicle may be useful if moving the patient over long distances depending on the terrain. Also, if you have a way to drag the sled other than manpower (e.g., dog, motor sled), it can save a lot of energy.

There are many ways this can be constructed. If you have a pair of skis, they can come in very handy. Ensure the patient is well secured, and attach a means of dragging the sled, e.g., rope.

Here are some examples:

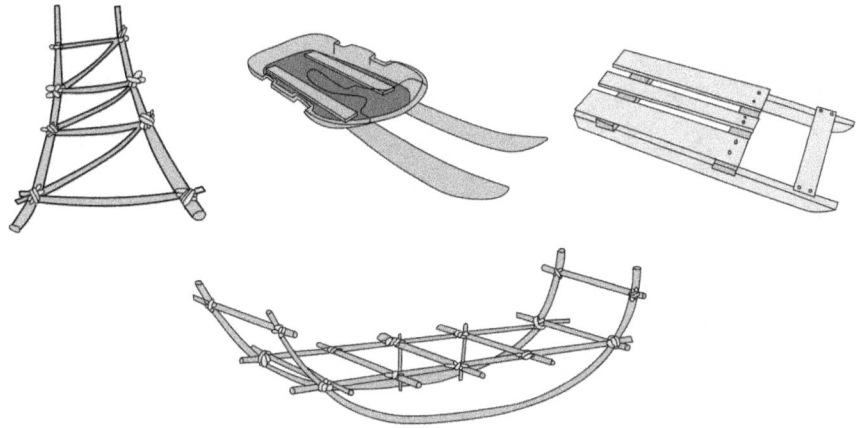

PART TWO: DIAGNOSIS & TREATMENTS

ENVIRONMENTALLY INDUCED

ALTITUDE INDUCED

There are a variety of conditions that can occur when going into high altitudes, and as with most things, prevention is the best option.

Only a few of the more severe and/or more common conditions are detailed here. As a 'cure-all,' if someone gets sick and you can't figure it out, you should descend.

GENERAL PREVENTION OF ALTITUDE-INDUCED ILLNESSES

Do not consume alcohol.

Maintain adequate hydration and nutrition (a 70% carbohydrate diet may help).

Take the time to acclimatize.

Train for endurance and strength before going to high elevations.

Acclimatizing to Altitude

Make day trips to a higher altitude with a return to lower altitude for sleep.

Mild exercise may be helpful, but extreme exercise may have the opposite effect.

Above 3,000 m (10,000 ft.), ascend no more than 1000 m (3000 ft.) in a 24-hour period, and have a rest day. Rest every 2 to 3 days.

Acetazolamide can be taken 24 hours before and during the ascent until acclimatization has occurred, which is usually after 48 hours at the maximum altitude.

Dexamethasone is another option for those that can't take acetazolamide, but it has a greater chance of causing side effects.

Ibuprofen may help. Administer until the highest altitude is attained for 48 hours.

ACUTE MOUNTAIN SICKNESS (AMS)

Rapid change in elevation may cause a condition known as altitude sickness or acute mountain sickness (AMS).

AMS occurs most commonly when approaching 2,400 m (8000 ft.) above sea level although there are many cases of AMS occurring at lower altitudes. It is usually aggravated by exertion.

Symptoms of AMS

Mild AMS most commonly occurs at altitudes over 2,500 m (8000 ft.).

Symptoms are similar to being hungover and include:

- Dizziness
- Headache (often precluding AMS)
- Increased heart rate
- Insomnia
- Fatigue
- Lack of appetite
- Nausea
- Pins and needles/tingling
- Shortness of breath
- Vomiting

Symptoms of Severe AMS

- Chest congestion
- Confusion
- Cough that may produce blood and/or phlegm
- Cyanosis (blue, gray, or purple discoloration of the skin)
- Dehydration
- Indifferent behavior
- Loss of coordination

- Unconsciousness

Treatment for AMS

- Avoid narcotics
- Maintain hydration and nutrition
- Stop ascending
- Descend if symptoms do not dissipate after 24 hours
- Acetazolamide: 200 mg orally every 8 hours, maximum 1 gram/day
- Dexamethasone: 3 mg ever 8 hours
- Nausea medications

HAPE AND HACE

High-altitude pulmonary edema (HAPE) and high-altitude cerebral edema (HACE) occur when the high altitude causes edema in the lungs (pulmonary) or brain (cerebral).

Edema is basically an accumulation of fluid resulting in swelling.

Both HAPE and HACE can be life threatening, and they can occur together. Treatment for both is the same.

Symptoms of HAPE

- Cough: Mild and dry at onset and becoming more productive in later stages
- Cyanosis (blue, gray, or purple discoloration of the skin)
- Increased pulse and respiratory rate
- Fatigue
- Fluid in lungs resulting in a gurgling sound (rales)
- Mild fever
- Shortness of breath
- Weakness

Symptoms of HACE

- Confusion
- Decreased consciousness
- Hallucinations (rare)
- Lethargy
- Seizures (rare)
- Severe headache
- Vomiting

Treatment for HAPE and HACE

- Descend as much as possible, at least 500 m.
- PROP
- Consider hyperbaric bag, preferably after descent.
- Acetazolamide: Every 8 to 12 hours, reduce dosage as symptoms decline.
- Dexamethasone: 4 mg every 6 hours until at safe elevation.
- Nifedipine (Procardia): for HAPE, 20 mg every 6 to 8 hours. **Note:** Will lower blood pressure.
- Sildenafil (Viagra): Helps to treat HAPE.
- Inhaled beta-agonists, e.g., Salmetero: Helps to treat HAPE.

Prevention of HAPE and HACE

- Acetazolamide: Start a couple of days before the planned ascent.
- Dexamethasone: HAPE preventative, 4 mg every 12 hours.
- Nifedipine (Procardia): HAPE preventative, 20 mg every 6 to 8 hours. **Note:** Will lower blood pressure.
- Sildenafil (Viagra): HAPE preventative
- Inhaled beta-agonists, e.g., Salmetero: HAPE preventative
- Ginkgo biloba

Related Chapters

- Diagnosis and Treatments > Head > Brain
- Must Read > Immediate First Aid > Critical First Aid > Breathing

HAFE

High-altitude flatus expulsion (HAFE) is the occurrence of flatulence as a result of high altitude. It is an inconvenience but generally harmless.

Treatment for HAFE

- Carbohydrate diet
- Descent
- Simethicone: 80 mg.

HIGH-ALTITUDE PHARYNGITIS AND BRONCHITIS

High-altitude pharyngitis and bronchitis usually occur at over 2,400 m (8000 ft.) of elevation.

Symptoms of High-Altitude Pharyngitis and Bronchitis

- Chronic cough which can be either dry or productive
- Dry or cracking nasal passages
- Reddened and painful throat

Treatment for High-Altitude Pharyngitis and Bronchitis

- Hydration
- Lozenges or hard candies
- Nasal saline spray
- Steam inhalation
- Albuterol (common asthma medication)

PERIPHERAL EDEMA

Peripheral edema is swelling of the soft tissues, usually in hands, face, and ankles.

Treatment for Peripheral Edema

- Will self-resolve when patient is acclimatized.
- Examine for AMS, HAPE, or HACE.
- Acetazolamide: 125 to 250 mg.

Related Chapters

- Diagnosis and Treatments > Environmentally Induced > Altitude Induced

ANIMALS: MARINE

GENERAL TREATMENTS

Specifics depending on the creature are given, but for ease of memory and in case the cause is unknown, here are some general diagnoses and treatments.

MARINE TOXINS

These include stings from jellyfish, corals, and anemones.

General Symptoms of Marine Toxins

- Local pain
- Swelling
- Tenderness

General Treatment for Marine Toxins

- Do not rub/scrape.
- Topical decontaminant, e.g., vinegar
- If decontaminant is more than two minutes away, rinse wound with seawater and then apply decontaminant when available.
- If seawater is not available, use fresh water very forcefully.
- Remove nematocysts.
- Shave site. Be sure to use shaving cream or similar.
- Treat wound.

Related Chapters

- Must Read > Open Wounds, Skin Infections, and Sepsis > Open Wounds

SPINY INJURIES

These come from marine life such as stingrays, catfish, stonefish, etc.

General Symptoms of Marine Spiny Injuries

- Puncture wounds
- Severe pain
- Tenderness
- Possible systemic symptoms

General Treatment for Marine Spiny Injuries

- Soak in water as hot as you can tolerate for about an hour or until relief.
- Remove any spine fragments during soak.
- Treat wound.

Related Chapters

- Must Read > Open Wounds, Skin Infections, and Sepsis > Open Wounds

BARRACUDA

Barracuda are large saltwater fish that can grow up to 2 m in length.

They are found in tropical and subtropical oceans all around the world, especially near coral reefs and near the top of the water.

They are not usually dangerous to humans, but their bite can cause a nasty wound.

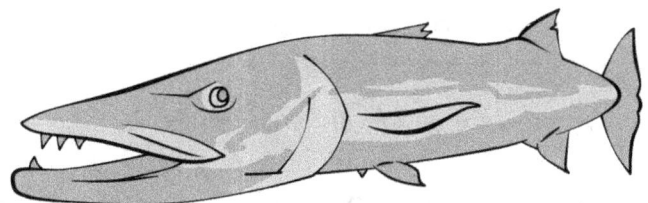

Treatment for a Barracuda Bite

- Treat wound.

Related Chapters

- Must Read > Open Wounds, Skin Infections, and Sepsis > Open Wounds

BLUE-RINGED OCTOPUS

The blue-ringed octopus is a relatively small octopus characterized by yellowish skin and blue and black rings.

When agitated, the brown patches will darken and pulsating blue rings or clumps will appear.

Although they are most commonly found in northern parts of Western Australia, New South Wales, and South Australia, they are also present in the eastern Indo-Pacific up to Japan. They enjoy tide pools and coral reefs in shallow coastal waters.

The blue-ringed octopus injects its victims with a cocktail of venoms, one of which is the paralytic tetrodotoxin; it is thought that it may be possible to feel minor effects of the envenomation even without being bitten, i.e., just by being near it.

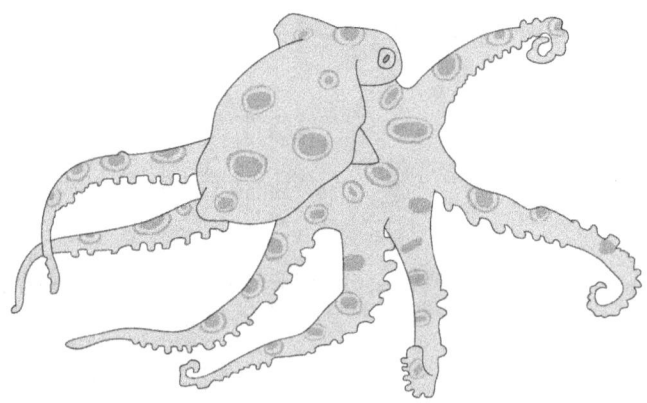

Symptoms of Blue-Ringed Octopus Envenomation

Initial:

- Minimal or no discomfort
- Small laceration with very minimal blood
- Little or no discoloration

Within ten minutes:

- Difficulty breathing
- Difficulty speaking
- Difficulty swallowing
- Nausea and vomiting
- Numbness
- Paresthesia (tingling)
- Progressive muscular weakness
- Visual disturbances

In severe cases:

- Cerebral anoxia (deficiency of oxygen in the brain tissue)
- Paralysis
- Respiratory failure

Treatment for Blue-ringed Octopus Envenomation

- Apply pressure-immobilization bandaging.
- Perform rescue breathing.

The patient will go into respiratory failure, but the effects of the venom will subside after some hours. Rescue breathing must be continued until the patient regains the ability to breathe on his/her own.

Related Chapters

- Must Read > Immediate First Aid > Pressure-Immobilization Technique
- Must Read > Immediate First Aid > Critical First Aid > Airway

BRISTLE-WORM

Bristle-worms are segmented worms with an elongated body. They can be as small as 3 cm or as large 60+ cm. They come in a variety of colors with the larger ones usually being brown or gray.

There are many types of bristle-worms, some of which have spines that, when handled, may dislodge into the skin.

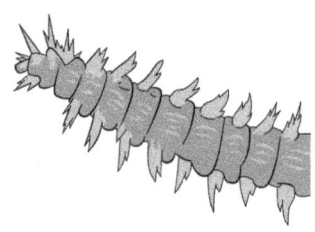

Symptoms of a Bristle-Worm Injury

- Burning sensation
- Flaking of the skin
- Itching
- Raised red rash
- Swelling in the soft tissue

Treatment for a Bristle-Worm Injury

- Remove large bristles with forceps.
- Dry the skin gently.
- Apply sticky adhesive tape and then peel off to remove embedded spines.
- Vinegar for 15 minutes will help soothe the pain.
- Topical corticosteroid: Apply a light layer.
- Systemic corticosteroid (e.g., prednisone) for severe cases

CATFISH

Catfish are found all over the world, and the venom is located in their fin-spines. Some even secrete toxin through their skin.

The ones that are most likely to sting humans are freshwater catfish and, to a lesser extent, those found amongst coral.

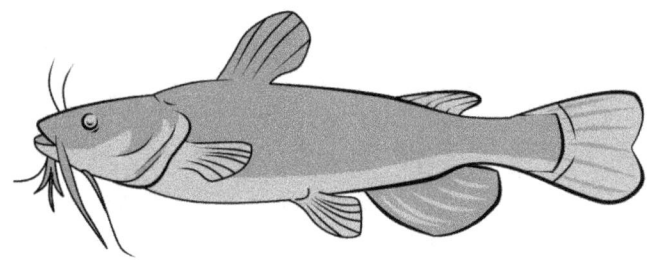

Symptoms of a Catfish Sting

- Cyanosis at sting site (blue, gray, or purple discoloration of the skin)
- Fainting
- General weakness
- Increased perspiration
- Involuntary muscle movement
- Low blood pressure
- Respiratory distress
- Scalding, stinging, or throbbing pain which can last up to 48 hours but generally dissipates within 60 minutes
- Swelling

Treatment for a Catfish Sting

- Soak in water as hot as you can tolerate for about an hour or until relief.

- Remove spine fragments during the soak.
- Treat wound.

Related Chapters

- Must Read > Open Wounds, Skin Infections, and Sepsis > Open Wounds

CONUS

Conus creatures encompass a range of predatory sea snails of various sizes found mainly in the tropics, e.g., cone shells, cone snails. All conus snails are venomous and use this venom to paralyze their prey by shooting dart-like teeth from their mouths.

Symptoms of Conus Envenomation

Initial:

- Cyanosis (blue, gray, or purple discoloration of the skin)
- Local numbness
- Mild sting

Advanced:

- Altered vision
- Difficulty swallowing
- Fainting
- Itching, tingling, tickling, pricking, or burning of skin
- Loss of neurologic reflexes, e.g., knee jerk reaction
- Nausea
- Voice loss
- Weakness
- Muscular paralysis
- Respiratory failure
- Cardiac failure
- Coma

Treatment for Conus Envenomation

- Pressure-immobilization technique

Related Chapters

- Must Read > Immediate First Aid > Pressure-Immobilization Technique

CORAL

Cuts and abrasions from corals may be a simple wound, but sometimes there may be toxins present.

Symptoms of Coral Toxin Contact

Initial reaction:

- Itching
- Redness
- Stinging pain

Followed by:

- General sick feeling
- Low-grade fever
- Red raised welts

Progressing:

- Skin infection
- Tissue sloughing (shedding of dead tissue)
- Ulceration

Treatment for Coral Toxin Contact

- Neutralize stinging with diluted vinegar (half-strength) followed by copious water irrigation.
- Treat as an open wound with aggressive cleaning and wet-to-dry dressings.

Related Chapters

- Must Read > Open Wounds, Skin Infections, and Sepsis > Open Wounds

JELLYFISH

Jellyfish sting with nematocysts, usually triggered by physical contact. Contact with a tentacle can cause many stinging cells to fire.

Anemones, fire coral, and hydroids all work in a similar way and are treated as such.

Due to the large variety of jellyfish, knowing which ones are venomous often requires local knowledge. The best thing to do is to stay away from all jellyfish.

Jellyfish-safe sunblock and stinger suits are also available in cases where entering infested waters is unavoidable.

Symptoms of Jellyfish Stings

There is a massive range of symptoms depending on the specific creature, and they span most of the body's functions.

Seeing the creature and/or recognizing it by the site of attack is the best indicator.

Local knowledge is needed.

Treatment for Jellyfish Stings

- Do not rub/scrape.
- Topical decontaminant, e.g., vinegar
- If decontaminant is more than 2 minutes away, rinse wound with seawater and then apply decontaminant when available.
- If seawater is not available, use freshwater very forcefully.
- Remove nematocysts.
- Shave site. Be sure to use shaving cream or similar.
- Corticosteroids

Treatment for serious reactions:

- Seek advanced medical care.
- Maintain the airway and administer oxygen.
- Treat anaphylaxis if needed.
- Try to identify species.

If there is eye damage:

- Irrigate with saline.
- Seek medical help.

Related Chapters

- Must Read > Immediate First Aid > Anaphylaxis

LEECHES

Leeches suck the blood of their hosts until they are full, then they fall off. It is usually painless and can go unnoticed.

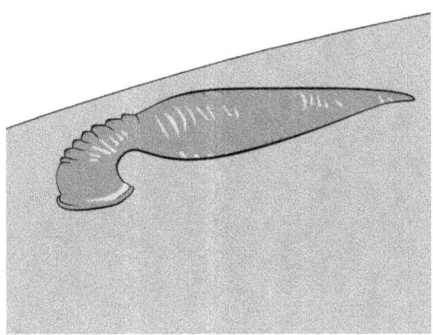

Symptoms of a Leech Bite

- Slow-healing, freely bleeding wound
- Possible allergic reaction, e.g., rash

Treatment for a Leech Bite

Removal:

- Do not rip off.
- Apply a few drops of alcohol or vinegar.
- Holding a flame near site may also help.

After removal:

- Inspect for retained mouthparts.
- Treat wound.
- Use a hemostatic.

Related Chapters

- Must Read > Open Wounds, Skin Infections, and Sepsis> Open Wounds

MORAY EEL

Morays have an extremely forceful bite which can cause severe puncture wounds. There are many different species, but the basic appearance is similar.

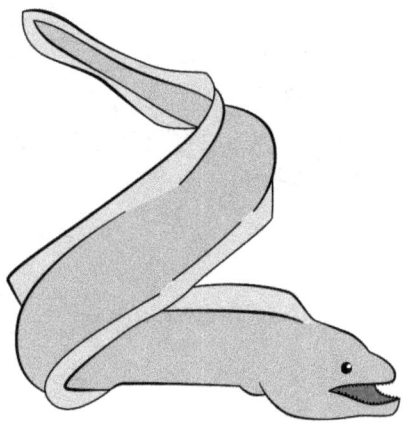

Treatment for Moray Eel Bite

- Treat as an open wound.

Related Chapters

- Must Read > Open Wounds, Skin Infections, and Sepsis > Open Wounds

SEA CUCUMBER

Sea cucumbers are found all over the world. They have an elongated body with leathery skin and produce a toxin in their tentacles.

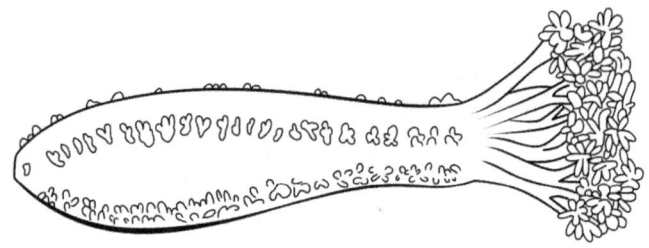

Symptoms of Sea Cucumber Toxin Contact

- Dermatitis
- Eye irritation
- Severe illness and possible death if toxin is ingested

Treatment for Sea Cucumber Toxin Contact

- Wash with soap and water.
- Topical detoxification, e.g., vinegar

If there is eye damage:

- Anesthetize.
- Irrigate.
- Seek advanced medical help.

SEA LION

A bite from a seal or sea lion will result in an infection known as seal finger. It can also result from any contact of an open wound (even very minor) with the animal's mouth, bones, or coat.

Symptoms of Seal Finger

- Pain
- Swelling of digits
- Taut, shiny skin

Treatment for Seal Finger

- Treat wound.
- Antibiotic: Tetracycline 1,500 mg initially, then 500 mg every 6 hours for 4 to 6 weeks.

Related Chapters

- Must Read > Open Wounds, Skin Infections, and Sepsis > Open Wounds

SEA SNAKE

Sea snakes are usually found in warm coastal waters from the Indian Ocean to the Pacific. They are closely related to venomous Australian snakes, and as such, many of them are very venomous. Fortunately, most bites do not result in envenomation.

Most sea snakes are completely aquatic, but some of them can come onto land.

Symptoms of Sea Snake Envenomation

Initial symptoms may not show for up to 8 hours.

Initial:

- Anxiety
- Euphoria
- Malaise (general unease)

After 30 to 60 minutes:

- Muscle aching and stiffness
- Dysarthria (difficulty in using speaking muscles)
- Sialorrhea (excessive salivation)

After 3 to 6 hours:

- Cyanosis (blue, gray, or purple discoloration of the skin)
- Dilated pupils
- Moderate to severe pain
- Muscle spasms, starting from the bottom and moving up
- Loss of vision (severe cases)
- Nausea
- Vomiting

Treatment for Sea Snake Envenomation

- Pressure-immobilization technique
- PROP
- Antivenin (anticipate anaphylaxis)

Related Chapters

- Must Read > Immediate First Aid > Pressure-Immobilization Technique
- Must Read > Immediate First Aid > Critical First Aid > Breathing
- Must Read > Immediate First Aid > Anaphylaxis

SEA URCHIN

Sea urchins are found in all oceans and come in a variety of colors.

They can envenomate their victims either via their spine or their pedicellariae (pincer-type organs).

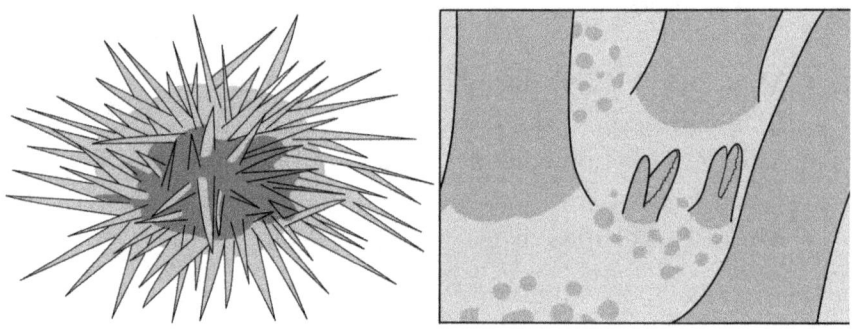

Symptoms of Sea Urchin Envenomation

- Aphonia (inability to speak or produce vocalizations)
- Black or purple markings
- Burning
- Dizziness
- Fainting
- Hypotension
- Joint pain
- Malaise (general unease)
- Muscle aching
- Muscular paralysis
- Pain (intense)
- Redness
- Respiratory distress
- Swelling
- Weakness

Treatment for Sea Urchin Envenomation

- Soak in water as hot as you can tolerate for about an hour or until relief.
- Remove spines.
- Splint if spines remain near a joint.
- If pedicellariae are attached, apply shaving foam and scrape them away with a razor.

SHARKS

Sharks are found in all oceans and come in a range of shapes, sizes, and aggressiveness.

Treatment for a Shark Bite

- Treat wound.
- Abrasions from contact with the shark's skin should be treated as a burn.

Related Chapters

- Must Read > Open Wounds, Skin Infections, and Sepsis > Open Wounds
- Diagnosis and Treatments > Environmentally Induced > Heat and/or Sun Induced > Burns

SPINE FISH

This covers all fish that envenomate via spines, e.g., leatherbacks, lionfish (left picture), ratfish, toadfish, scorpion fish, and stonefish (right picture).

Different fish inflict different levels of envenomation. Stonefish are generally considered the most venomous and cause the most pain, which can be excruciating.

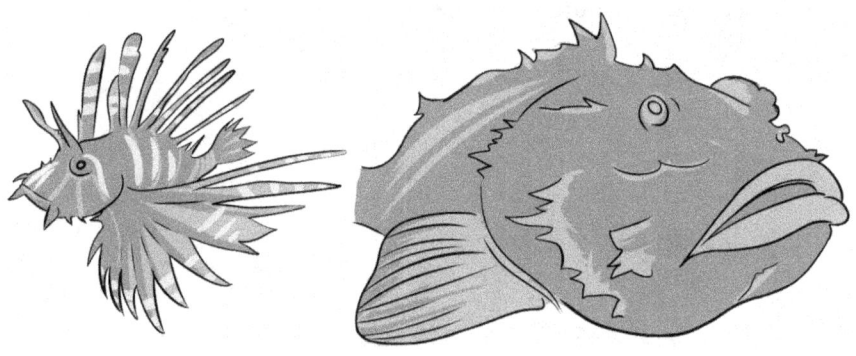

Symptoms of Spine Fish Envenomation

- Immediate, intense pain, peaking at about 1 to 2 hours and lasting for up to 12 hours
- Blisters
- Bruising
- Numbness
- Redness
- Swelling
- Tissue shedding

Many other symptoms may occur depending on the exact species including gastrointestinal problems, paralysis, respiratory and/or cardiovascular failure, etc.

Treatment for Spine Fish Envenomation

- Soak in water as hot as you can tolerate for about an hour or until relief.
- Remove any spine fragments during soak.
- Antivenin (anticipate anaphylaxis)

Related Chapters

- Must Read > Immediate First Aid > Anaphylaxis

SPONGES

Sponges come in many different shapes, sizes, and colors. They are attached to the sea floor or coral beds and are full of pores which allow water to circulate through them. They also contain chemical toxins which can affect humans if touched. Even dry sponges may remain toxic, so do not handle them without gloves.

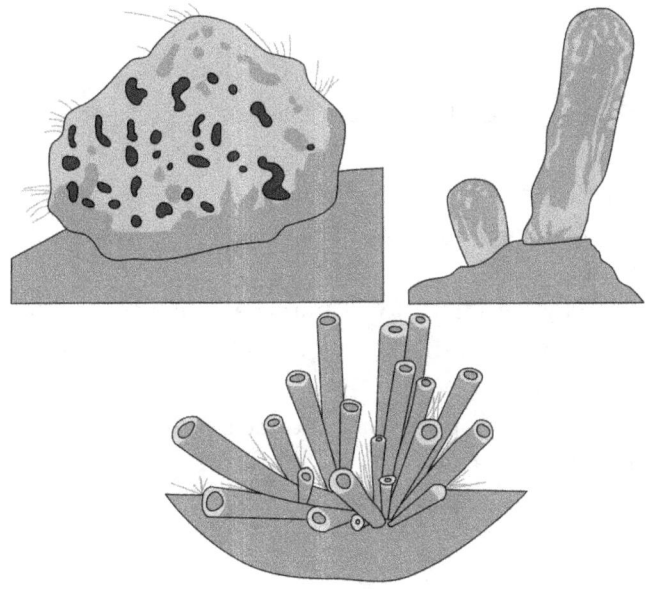

Symptoms of Sponge Toxin Contact

Minor:

- Blistering
- Burning sensation
- Itching
- Swelling at joints
- Stiffness at joints
- Minor reactions usually subside within 7 days, faster if treated.

Severe:

- Chills
- Dizziness
- General sick feeling
- Feeling like an insect is crawling on or under skin
- Fever
- Muscle cramps
- Nausea
- Skin peeling after 10 days

Treatment for Sponge Toxin Contact

- Gently dry the skin.
- Apply and remove sticky adhesive tape to remove adherent spicules.
- Soak in vinegar for 10 to 30 minutes, 3 or 4 times a day.
- Hydrocortisone or triamcinolone only after at least two vinegar soaks
- Corticosteroid: Topical for minor reactions and/or oral for severe reactions

STINGRAY

Stingrays are cartilaginous fish related to sharks and come in a variety of colors and sizes. If injured by a stingray sting, the patient may suffer a puncture/laceration as well as envenomation.

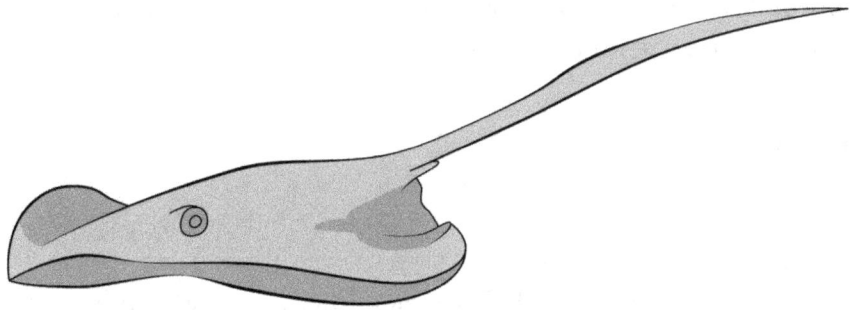

Symptoms of Stingray Envenomation

Local:

- Dusky discoloration
- Intense pain
- Redness of skin
- Swelling

Other

- Death of body tissue
- Fat and muscle hemorrhage
- Fainting
- Malaise (general sick feeling)
- Muscle cramps
- Paralysis
- Vertigo (perception of motion, usually spinning)

Treatment for Sting Ray Envenomation

- Soak in water as hot as you can tolerate for about an hour or until relief.
- Remove spine fragments, which can be done while soaking.

Note: If spine is deeply embedded, manage as impaling object; otherwise, treat as an open wound.

Related Chapters

- Must Read > Open Wounds, Skin Infections, and Sepsis > Impaling Objects
- Must Read > Open Wounds, Skin Infections, and Sepsis > Open Wounds

WEEVER FISH

The weever fish is found in the Eastern Atlantic Ocean, European coastal areas, and Mediterranean Sea. They are brown and have venomous spines on their first dorsal fins and gills.

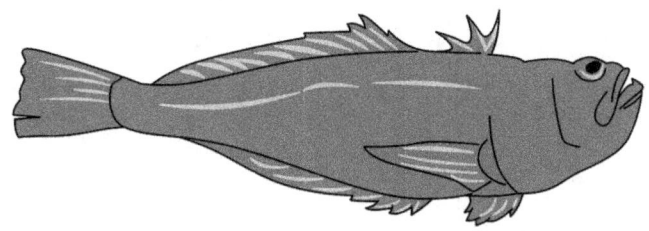

Symptoms of Weever Fish Envenomation

- Immediate intense pain (burning, crushing, or scalding) peaking at 30 minutes and lasting up to 72 hours
- Delirium
- Fainting
- Fever and chills
- Headache
- Irregular heart rate
- Nausea and/or vomiting
- Pale wound site, becoming red and warm after 8-ish hours
- Seizures
- Swelling, increasing for up to 10 days

Treatment for Weever Fish Envenomation

- Soak in water as hot as you can tolerate for about an hour or until relief.
- Remove any fragments, which can be done while soaking.
- Treat wound.

Related Chapters

- Must Read > Open Wounds, Skin Infections, and Sepsis > Open Wounds

ANIMALS: TERRESTRIAL

GENERAL PREVENTION OF ANIMAL ATTACK

- Leave animals alone.
- Do not feed, antagonize, or surprise them.
- Don't put your hands or feet in places you can't see; use sticks to turn over logs, rocks, etc.
- Don't try to take animals' food, block their escape, or get in between a mother and her offspring.
- Most animals are afraid of fire, loud noises, and humans in general.
- Wild animals are most dangerous when threatened, wounded, hungry, dehydrated, bearing young, etc.

If You Encounter Large Animals

- Keep calm, freeze, then slowly back away.
- Do not make any sudden movements.
- If the animal charges, move out of the way.
- If you need to run, do so in a zigzag pattern.
- Shouting and making a commotion may put off a predator.
- Climbing a tree is a last resort as the animal may wait for you.

ANT BITES

Fire ants often attack in mass if their nest is disturbed.

Treatment for Ant Bites

- Brush them away with your hand.
- Move away from the nest.
- Strip your clothes to ensure there are no ants inside them.
- Elevate the bitten extremity.
- Place a cool compress on the affected area.
- If a blister develops, don't pop it.
- If a blister pops, wash it with soap and water, then dress.
- Antihistamine
- Anti-inflammatory medication

BED BUGS

Bed bugs feed on your blood while you sleep and are most active at night. The bites are usually painless, but the after-effects vary.

Symptoms of Bed Bug Bites

- Resemble mosquito bites but often are multiple bites in a straight line.

Treatment for Bed Bug Bites

- Eradication
- Antihistamine
- Anti-inflammatory

Eradication of Bed Bugs

Find the nest: Check mattress seams, linens, backpacks, wooden joints, etc. Look for brown fecal markings and dried blood.

Once the nest has been found, there are a number of methods which can be used to eradicate bed bugs:

- Use bedding covers to starve them out although adult bed bugs can live for more than a year without a blood meal.
- Diatomaceous earth is a natural pesticide found at most organic gardening supply stores. Dust the seams of the mattress with it. Note: It won't kill the eggs.
- Extreme cold: 5 days of temperatures >15 °C (about 0 °F)
- Pesticides: Cover all areas and repeat at least once 10 days after the initial treatment.
- Placing all bedding and clothes in a hot dryer (as hot as possible) for 90 minutes.

- Rubbing alcohol: Apply and repeat for a week.
- Vacuum the flooring and upholstery: A stiff brush is helpful to scrub mattress seams before vacuuming.
- Wash in hot, soapy water over 50 °C (125 °F).

BEE/WASP STING

The sooner you treat a sting the better, but you should first leave the area to prevent further attack.

Treatment for Bee/Wasp Stings

- Remove the bee stinger with tweezers or by scraping it with a credit card or your fingernail. Be careful not to squeeze the venom from the sack into your body.
- Treat as an open wound.
- Antihistamine
- Ice topically to soothe.
- Mix baking soda with a small amount of water to form a paste and apply topically.
- Mud applied topically may soothe if nothing else is available.

Related Chapters

- Must Read > Open Wounds, Skin Infections, and Sepsis > Open Wounds

CATERPILLARS

Caterpillars are found all over the world and come in a large variety of sizes and colors. Some caterpillars have spines containing toxin.

Symptoms of Caterpillar Toxin Contact

From caterpillars with hollow spines and venom glands:

- Instant pain
- Redness
- Swelling

Systemic symptoms are rare but may occur. These include:

- Fever
- Headache
- Nausea and vomiting
- Swollen lymph nodes
- Impaired blood clotting (rare)

From caterpillars or moths:

- Conjunctivitis
- Itching
- Papular rash (an area of abnormal skin tissue that is less than 1 centimeter around)
- Redness
- Upper respiratory irritation

Treatment for Caterpillar Toxin Contact

- Apply and remove adhesive tape to remove spines.
- Antihistamine

- Anti-inflammatory
- Corticosteroid

CAT-SCRATCH DISEASE

Cat-scratch disease is, not surprisingly, most commonly caused by cat scratches, but dog and monkey bites can also transmit the disease, as can thorns and splinters.

Symptoms of Cat-Scratch Disease

- Chills
- Insect bite-like papule (solid elevation of skin with no visible fluid; can be brown, purple, pink, or red in color and varied in size)
- Mild fever
- Nausea
- Painful and tender lymph nodes, usually of arm or leg
- Rashes

Treatment for Cat-Scratch Disease

- Will usually self-resolve within months.
- Antibiotic: Ciprofloxacin 500 mg twice a day.

FLEAS

Fleas are tiny, wingless, blood-sucking external parasites. They suck the blood of birds and mammals, including humans.

Common areas for flea bites are ankles, armpits, breasts, groin, legs, underside of elbows, underside of knees, and waistline.

Symptoms of Flea Bites

- Hives
- Itchy
- Rash
- Red halo around bite
- Several small red bite bumps in groups or straight lines
- Soreness around bite

Treatment for Fleas Bites

- Flea bites will dissipate in time.
- Eradicate.
- Avoid scratching.
- Antihistamine

Eradication of Fleas

- Botanical dust mixed with a borate powder or boric acid. Do not breathe in. Coat the area and then vacuum after 24 hours.
- Insect growth regulator (IGR), e.g., Nylar
- Very fine salt: Coat the area and then vacuum after 24 hours.

INSECTS: GENERAL

Due to the incredible number of different insects, it is useful to have a general diagnosis and treatment for those you cannot identify easily.

Prevention is the best way to avoid attack. There are many insect repellents out there. If no insect repellents are available, you can use smoke to fumigate them.

General Symptoms of Insect Bites or Stings

There are a wide range of symptoms depending on the species. Common general symptoms include:

- Allergic reactions
- Pain
- Swelling
- Welts

For multiple stings:

- Diarrhea
- Respiratory distress
- Vomiting

Note: Even a single sting may bring on anaphylaxis, which is life threatening.

General Treatment for Insect Bites or Stings

- Treat critical systems as needed.
- Charcoal: Activated charcoal is preferable. If that is unavailable, mix tea and wood charcoal (not briquettes) and add milk of magnesia if available.

- Use a specific antidote/treatment if available/known.

Related Chapters

- Must Read > Immediate First Aid > Anaphylaxis

MAMMALIAN BITES

Apart from the obvious wound, other problems an animal bite can cause are the transfer of disease and a higher chance of infection than many other types of wounds. Rabies is a potentially fatal infection that can occur, as is tetanus.

Keep your vaccinations up to date.

Treatment for Mammalian Bites

Different animals carry different diseases, e.g., plague is carried by rats and fleas, whereas tuberculosis is usually associated with deer, elk, and bison. Regardless of what bites you encounter, initial field treatment is the same, even if bitten by a human.

- Remove any rings or bracelets that may get stuck if swelling occurs.
- Treat wound and clean thoroughly.

The antiseptic of choice is benzalkonium chloride (BZK) as it has some effect against rabies.

If over the next few weeks after being bitten there are any of the following symptoms, seek advanced medical care:

- Diarrhea
- Fever
- Nausea
- Vomiting

Related Chapters

- Diagnosis and Treatments > Musculoskeletal System > Tetanus

- Must Read > Open Wounds, Skin Infections, and Sepsis > Open Wounds
- Diagnosis and Treatments > Environmentally Induced > Animals: Terrestrial > Mammalian Bites > Rabies

RABIES

Rabies is a fatal viral disease which any mammal can contract. Bats, cats, cattle, dogs, foxes, monkeys, raccoons, skunks, and wolves are the greatest risk to humans. Vaccinations are available.

Symptoms of Rabies

Symptoms in rabies victims are usually delayed for about 30 days. After this symptom-free period, victims may experience:

- Fatigue
- Fever
- Headache
- Loss of appetite

Increased symptoms

- Irritability
- Disorientation
- Hallucination
- Seizures
- Eventual paralysis, coma, cardiac arrest, or respiratory failure

Treatment for Rabies

Once symptoms start to show, chances of survival are slim.

- Immediately treat wound after any possible exposure, e.g., when bitten.
- Seek advanced medical care.

If animal saliva has come in contact with your eye, irrigate it well with water and seek advanced medical care.

MOSQUITOES

Mosquitoes are found all over the world. Usually their bite results in nothing more than itchiness and minor swelling. For some people the symptoms can be a bit worse, e.g., hives. Unfortunately, mosquitoes also transmit a number of potentially deadly diseases.

Prevention of Mosquito Bites

- Avoid mosquito-infested areas. They are attracted to standing water and moist areas and are most active at dusk and dawn.
- Keep up to date on all relevant immunizations, especially if traveling to at-risk countries.
- Wear long clothing and insect repellant; if no insect repellents are available, you can use smoke to fumigate clothing.

Related Chapters

- Must Read > Prevention > Vaccinations

DENGUE FEVER

Dengue fever is a tropical disease.

Symptoms of Dengue Fever

- Diarrhea
- Fever
- Headache
- Muscle and joint pains
- Skin rash akin to measles
- Vomiting

Symptoms of dengue hemorrhagic fever:

- Bruising and bleeding from the gums, mouth, and nose

Treatment for Dengue Fever

There is no specific antiviral drug for dengue fever, and complete recovery can take up to a month.

- Treat dehydration.
- Treat symptoms.

Related Chapters

- Diagnosis and Treatments > Circulatory System > Dehydration and Volume Shock

JAPANESE ENCEPHALITIS

Japanese encephalitis occurs all year round in tropical and subtropical areas and during the warmer months in temperate climates.

Vaccinations are available and recommended if visiting high-risk countries, especially in rural areas.

Symptoms of Japanese Encephalitis

Less than 1% of people infected will become ill. This means that in most cases, no symptoms will show.

Symptoms that may develop:

- Chills
- Fatigue
- Fever
- Headache
- Nausea
- Vomiting

Severe symptoms of Japanese Encephalitis:

Encephalitis (inflammation of the brain) develops in about 1 in 300 infections.

- Coma
- Paralysis
- Seizures

Treatment for Japanese Encephalitis

There is no specific treatment.

- Treat dehydration.
- Treat symptoms.

Related Chapters

- Must Read > Prevention > Vaccinations
- Diagnosis and Treatments > Circulatory System > Dehydration and Volume Shock

MALARIA

Malaria prophylaxis (prevention) medications are available and recommended if visiting high-risk countries, especially rural areas. There are many types to suit different needs, e.g., dosages per day, short versus long-term travel, various strains, etc.

An antibiotic recommended in the first aid kit that can also double as a malaria prophylactic is doxycycline.

Dosage for doxycycline as a malaria prophylactic:

- 100 mg once a day
- Start a couple of days before exposure (travel to endemic area).
- Continue daily during exposure.
- Continue for 4 weeks after exposure.
- Do not exceed 4 months of medication, i.e., only stay in the exposed area for three months.

Symptoms of Malaria

- Confusion
- Fever and chills that are recurring
- Flu-like symptoms that do not respond to normal treatments
- Headaches
- Jaundice (yellow coloring of the skin and eyes)
- Muscle pain
- Nausea
- Respiratory difficulties
- Tiredness
- Vomiting

Treatment for Malaria

- Seek advanced medical care.
- Keep well hydrated.
- Avoid NSAIDs, but acetaminophen may help.
- Antibiotic: Doxycycline 100 mg twice a day for 7 days.

Note: Depending on the strain of malaria, doxycycline may need to be used in combination with other medications. If you suspect you have malaria, seek advanced medical care for definite diagnosis and treatment.

Related Chapters

- First Aid Kit

WEST NILE VIRUS

West Nile virus is found in temperate and tropical regions of the world.

Symptoms of West Nile Virus

The majority of people will not have any symptoms, but 20% of infected people may have the following:

- Difficulty concentrating
- Fatigue
- Fever
- Headache
- Nausea and vomiting
- Rash
- Swollen lymph nodes

Under 1% of infected people may develop encephalitis or meningitis.

Treatment for West Nile Virus

No specific treatment is available, but it will usually self-resolve within a few days.

- Treat symptoms.
- Seek advanced medical care if you experience altered mental state, severe headaches, and/or stiff neck.

Related Chapters

- Diagnosis and Treatments > Head > Brain > Meningitis

YELLOW FEVER

Yellow fever is most common in areas of Africa and South America. It mostly affects the liver and can be deadly.

Vaccinations are available and recommended if visiting high-risk countries, especially rural areas.

Symptoms of Yellow Fever

Mild:

- Usually dissipate within days.
- Dizziness
- Fever
- Headache
- Loss of appetite
- Muscle aches, particularly in your back and knees
- Nausea and/or vomiting
- Red eyes, face, or tongue
- Sensitivity to light

Severe:

The mild symptoms may return and also bring other symptoms which may be fatal.

- Abdominal pain
- Bleeding from your nose, mouth, and eyes
- Brain dysfunction
- Decreased urination
- Jaundice (yellow coloring of the skin and eyes)
- Liver and kidney failure
- Vomiting, sometimes of blood

Treatment for Yellow Fever

There is no specific treatment for yellow fever.

- Treat symptoms.
- Seek advanced medical care.
- Avoid NSAIDs.

Related Chapters

- Must Read > Prevention > Vaccinations

CUTANEOUS MYIASIS

Cutaneous myiasis occurs when certain fly species lay eggs on the skin which then hatch and larvae enter the skin.

Symptoms of Cutaneous Myiasis

- Feeling of something under the skin
- Fever (rare)
- Pain
- Lesions
- Swollen lymph nodes (rare)

Treatment for Cutaneous Myiasis

- Simple pressure may force it out.
- Covering the breathing hole with animal fat or nail polish may cause the larvae to emerge.
- If that does not work, inject 2 ml of local anesthetic (if available) into the base of the lesion to force them out with pressure.
- If that does not work or anesthetic is unavailable, cut the larvae out, ensuring they do not rupture.

MITES AND CHIGGERS

Chiggers are a type of mite found all over the world that favor moist and/or green areas, e.g., gardens, forests, and parks.

They are extremely small red creatures that are best seen with a magnifying glass and/or when they are in groups.

Prevention is the same as for mosquitoes.

For other mite bites, see scabies.

Symptoms of Chigger Bites

- Extreme itchiness
- Bites are red and may be flat, raised, or blister-like.
- Usually occur in the folds of the skin, e.g., armpits or behind knees.

Treatment for Chigger Bites

- Chiggers do not cause any diseases and will go away on their own.
- Itching will last for several days, lesions up to 14 days.
- Avoid hot water, e.g., baths and showers.
- Do not scratch.
- They do not burrow into the skin, so there is no need to try to remove them.
- Treat itching and inflammation.
- Antihistamine
- Calamine lotion
- Corticosteroid creams

Scabies is caused by mites that burrow into the skin. These mites cause an allergic reaction resulting in extreme itchiness. Scabies itself is not contagious, but the passing of mites is via close skin contact, sharing of towels, etc.

Symptoms of Scabies Bites

- Bites are most commonly found on the armpits, buttocks, fingers, genitals of men, navel, outside of elbow, waistline, wrist (palm side), and sides of breasts in women.
- Rash with tiny blisters/sores
- Severe itching, worsening at night

Treatment for Scabies Bites

- Treat all people and clean at the same time to prevent reoccurrences.
- Clean clothing and linen well as you would for bedbugs.
- Apply Permethrin cream on bites and under the fingernails.

Related Chapters

- Diagnosis and Treatments > Environmentally Induced > Animals: Terrestrial > Mosquitoes
- Diagnosis and Treatments > Environmentally Induced > Animals: Terrestrial > Bed Bugs

PORCUPINES

Porcupines are rodents with sharp quills. They are found in Africa, the Americas, Europe, and Southern Asia.

Porcupine Quill Removal and Treatment

- The sooner they are removed the easier it will be.
- Do not cut them before removal.
- Pull them straight out from the base, along the same line they entered.
- Ensure there are no fragments left in the skin.
- If quills are deeply embedded, a small nick in the skin can be made to allow the barb to be extracted.
- Treat the wound.
- Consider rabies vaccine.

Related Chapters

- Must Read > Open Wounds, Skin Infections, and Sepsis > Open Wounds
- Diagnosis and Treatments > Environmentally Induced > Animals: Terrestrial > Mammalian Bites > Rabies

SCORPIONS

Scorpions have pincers which can hurt, but only the tail injects venom. The venom usually affects the nervous system.

Symptoms of Scorpion Sting

- Difficulty swallowing
- Increased saliva output
- Irritability
- Pain, numbness, and/or tingling in the area of the sting
- Rapid breathing and heart rate
- Restlessness or twitching
- Sweating
- Weakness

Treatment for Scorpion Sting

- Remove jewelry from the affected limb (swelling may occur).
- Wash the area with soap and water.
- Antihistamine
- Antivenin (anticipate anaphylaxis)

Related Chapters

- Must Read > Immediate First Aid > Anaphylaxis

SNAKES

There are many kinds of snakes in the world. Some are harmless while others may be deadly.

The best practice is to steer clear of all snakes unless you have sufficient information about local subspecies.

Symptoms of Snake Bite

- Exact symptoms vary and depend on the species.
- Pain at bite site
- Puncture wounds from fangs

Treatment for Snake Bite

Snake bite treatment revolves around minimizing tissue damage, reducing the effects of venom, and preventing further complications, e.g., anaphylaxis and respiratory distress.

- Be prepared for anaphylaxis, infection, respiratory distress, and other complications.
- Do not attempt to kill or capture the snake.
- Remove any constrictive items from the bitten limb in anticipation of swelling.
- Immobilize bitten extremity with splinting.
- The pressure-immobilization technique is recommended only for Australian snakes, cobra snakes, coral snakes, mamba snakes, and any other neuro-toxic snake envenomation.
- Avoid movement.
- Do not elevate limb.
- Hydrate.
- Seek advanced medical care.
- No NSAID's. Other analgesics may help.

- Antibiotics if advanced medical care is more than 5 hours away.
- Antibiotic: Cephalexin for 7 to 10 days.
- Antibiotic: Dicloxacillin for 7 to 10 days.

Related Chapters

- Must Read > Immediate First Aid > Pressure Immobilization Technique

SPIDER BITE

There are many different types of spiders, and many of their bites have no specific treatment.

Most cases will resolve themselves after a few days, but some spiders are venomous and their bites may lead to death if untreated.

General Symptoms of Spider Bites

The effects from non-toxic spider bites usually don't last for more than a few hours, but they may occasionally last for a few days.

- Blisters
- Immediate pain
- Rash and/or redness
- Swelling
- Two small puncture wounds

General Treatment for Spider Bites

- Wash well
- Rest
- Treat symptoms

Note: In the case of the Australian funnel-web spider, use the pressure-immobilization technique.

When to Seek Advanced Medical Care:

- Bitten by a known toxic species, e.g., brown recluse or black widow
- Intense pain
- Local symptoms last more than 24 hours.
- Systemic symptoms emerge

Aspirin: Mix with water to make a paste and apply it topically.

Baking soda: Mix with water to make a paste and apply it topically.

Basil: Crush dried basil to a fine dust and apply it topically.

Charcoal: Use as a poultice. Activated charcoal is preferable. If that is unavailable, mix tea and wood charcoal (not briquettes) and add milk of magnesia if available.

Related Chapter

- Must Read > Immediate First Aid > Pressure-Immobilization Technique

TICKS

Different breeds of ticks can transmit a number of different diseases, but prevention is basically the same, i.e., keep the ticks off you.

Ticks must be implanted on humans for at least 24 hours to transmit bacteria.

Tick Removal

- Pulling ticks off with tweezers is the preferred method.
- Grab the tick as close to your skin as you can.
- Pull the tick straight up and try to get all of it.
- Disinfect the area.

Other methods include:

- Smothering it with petroleum jelly.
- Lighting it on fire, although the patient may also get burned.

Prevention of Ticks

- Light-colored clothing that covers whole body, e.g., long sleeves
- Regular checks, at least once a day
- Stay away from common tick-infested areas, e.g., leaf litter, shaded woodpiles, and shrubs along game trails.
- Repellents, e.g., DEET (<35%), Picardin etc.
- Plants that repel ticks, e.g., eucalyptus, garlic, lavender, mint, and sage (rub the leaves on your skin)

LYME DISEASE

Lyme disease is spread by the black-legged tick (deer tick).

Symptoms of Lyme Disease

Initial:

- Fatigue
- Fever
- Headache
- Joint pain
- Red rash around site

After weeks or months:

- Arthritis
- Infection
- Meningitis
- Neurological issues
- Rash

Treatment for Lyme Disease

- Antibiotic: Doxycycline 100 mg orally every 12 hours for 28 days.
- Antibiotics, other: Amoxicillin, azithromycin, and tetracycline

Related Chapters

- Diagnosis and Treatments > Head > Brain > Meningitis

ROCKY MOUNTAIN SPOTTED FEVER

Rocky Mountain spotted fever is a tick-transmitted disease spread by dog ticks.

Symptoms of Rocky Mountain Spotted Fever

Initial:

- Fever
- Headache
- Light sensitivity

After 3 to 4 days:

- High fever
- Rash

Treatment for Rocky Mountain Spotted Fever

- Antibiotic: Doxycycline 100 mg every 12 hours until 3 days after the fever subsides, usually 7 to 14 days.

TICK PARALYSIS

Symptoms of tick paralysis become present within 2 to 7 days of the tick(s) being attached.

Symptoms of Tick Paralysis

- Leg weakness
- Paralysis that travels up the trunk to the rest of the body
- Respiratory arrest

Treatment for Tick Paralysis

- Removal of the tick(s) will stop the toxin from being transferred into the body, and symptoms usually diminish quite quickly.
- Antibiotics can be used if you get a rash along with flu-like symptoms that are resistant to medicines.
- Antibiotic: Doxycycline 100 mg 2 times a day for 14 days.
- Antibiotic: Amoxicillin 500 mg 3 times a day for 14 days.
- Muscle aches and fatigue can linger for a while after treatment.

LICE

There are basically three types of lice: head, body, and pubic. They are most commonly spread through close contact and the sharing of personal items such as pillows, combs, towels, etc.

Lice can transmit disease (depending on the type), but they are species specific, i.e., a human cannot get lice from anything other than another human.

The best protection against all types of lice is good hygiene. When in unhygienic situations, check for lice as part of your daily hygiene routine.

Eradication of Lice

It is preferable to throw out or destroy (burn) anything that might be infested. If you cannot/do not want to destroy or throw it out, you have a few other options:

- Alcohol: Soak the infected items in strong alcohol.
- Hot water: Wash the infected items in very hot water.

- Suffocation: Place the infected items in plastic bags to suffocate the lice, and then air them out outside. Suffocate for two weeks, or five weeks for body lice.

Related Chapters

- Must Read > Prevention > Personal Hygiene

HEAD LICE

Head lice cause itching and sometimes a rash, but they do not carry disease.

Symptoms of Head Lice

- Itching
- Rash
- The nits (louse eggs) look like small bits of dandruff that stick to your hair. They are easily seen under a black light.

Treatment for Head Lice

- Eradication
- Run a fine tooth comb through the hair.
- Olive oil may be applied to the comb, which may make the nits easier to remove.

Wash hair with medicated shampoo:

- Start with dry hair.
- If you use hair conditioners, stop for a few days before using the medicine.
- Apply medicated shampoo to the hair and scalp.
- Let sit for 10 minutes, then rinse.
- Check with the comb after 8 and 12 hours.
- Repeat the process in 7 days.
- Change clothes daily if possible.

Medicated shampoos:

- Nix lotion (1% Permethrin) will kill both the lice and their eggs.

- Rid shampoo (Pyrethrum) will kill the lice but not their eggs.
- Kwell shampoo (Lindane) is much stronger and may cause neurological side effects in children.
- Various natural shampoos are also available.

PUBIC LICE

Pubic lice (crabs) may be either lice or mites. Although they usually start in the pubic hair, they can extend anywhere there is hair.

The infestation is usually passed by sexual contact and is not prevented with a condom.

Symptoms of Pubic Lice

- Severe itching

Treatment for Pubic Lice

- Use same treatment as for head lice.

BODY LICE

Body lice actually live on dirty clothes (especially the seams) as opposed to the body. They only go to the human body to feed and can live without a host for about a month.

Body lice carry infectious diseases.

Treatment for Body Lice

- Eradication
- Removal of the infested clothing. Destruction of the infested clothing is strongly advised.

COLD AND/OR WATER INDUCED

COLD is an acronym you can use to help you remember the prevention techniques for cold illnesses.

- **Cover** your extremities, i.e., head, hands (mittens work better than gloves), and feet.
- **Overexertion** will cause you to sweat, which will make your clothes wet, which will make you colder.
- **Layering:** Layers of loose-fitting lightweight clothing are a really good way to insulate your body. Wool and silk inner layers are better than cotton.
- **Dry:** Keep as dry as you can.

COLD WATER IMMERSION

Cold water immersion does not lead to immediate hypothermia. In fact, there are four phases of cold water immersion:

1. Cold shock response: This is the most common cause of drowning in cold water. It can cause a number of life-threatening conditions:

- **Gasp reflex:** When cold water is first entered, it causes an automatic gasp reflex. This reflex usually lasts about a minute, but if the head is under water at the time, it will lead to drowning.
- **Hyperventilation:** Panic can cause hyperventilation, which can lead to fainting, which can lead to drowning.
- **Cardiac arrest:** Vasoconstriction (narrowing of the arteries) means the heart must work harder.

2. Cold incapacitation. Prolonged vasoconstriction will cause the extremities to 'shut down,' which means the limbs will not be able to help keep the body afloat. This happens after about 10 minutes in the water.

3. Hypothermia. Hypothermia will set in after about 30 minutes in ice water for most adults.

4. Circum-rescue collapse. When a patient knows they are being rescued, their mental state relaxes. Blood pressure drops, muscles fail, and the patient may experience cardiac arrest. It can happen just before, during, or just after rescue.

Treatment for Cold Water Immersion

- Only enter water for rescue as a last resort.
- Exit the water slowly.

- Use in-water rescue breathing if needed.
- Treat critical systems as needed, e.g., CPR for cardiac arrest, treatment of hypothermia, etc.
- Start with 5 rescue breaths, and then continue as normal.
- If patient is breathing but unconscious, position them on his/her side.

Prevention of Cold Water Immersion

- Enter cold water slowly, keeping the head above the water.
- Wear a personal flotation device (PFD). These are designed to help keep the head above water, and they also provide warmth.
- Wear clothing to provide insulation.

If in the water:

- Assume the HELP (heat escape lessening position) (left picture) or huddle position (right picture) if in a group, placing children in the middle.

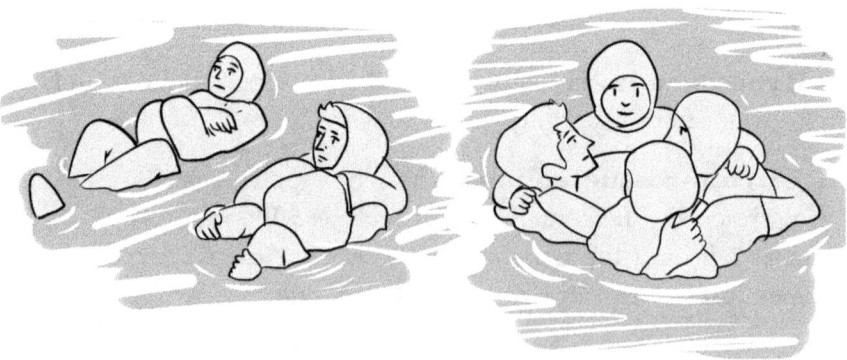

- Consider swimming to safety. The average person wearing a PFD can swim about 800 m in 10 °C water before failure.
- Control hyperventilation with controlled breathing.
- Tighten drawstrings.

Related Chapters

- Environmentally Induced > Cold and/or Water Induced > Hypothermia
- Must Read > Immediate First Aid > Critical First Aid > Airway

DROWNING

There are three basic classifications of drowning: Asymptomatic, symptomatic, and respiratory or cardiopulmonary arrest.

Symptoms of Asymptomatic Drowning

- The patient has been rescued from the water.
- Alert
- No respiratory distress
- With or without coughing

Treatment for Asymptomatic Drowning

- Monitor for respiratory symptoms.
- If respiratory symptoms develop, seek advanced medical care ASAP.
- Protect against and assess for hypothermia.
- Patients that do not worsen after 15 minutes are not likely to diminish but should still be monitored.

Symptoms of Symptomatic Drowning

- Patient requires resuscitation or shows signs of distress.

Treatment for Symptomatic Drowning

- Seek advanced medical care.
- Treat for respiratory or cardiopulmonary arrest. If the patient is still in the water, only use rescue breathing.

Prevention of Drowning

- Abandon a stalled vehicle in a flood area.
- Always wear a PFD in open water.
- Be prepared for flash flooding during heavy rainfall and seek high ground.
- Do not attempt a water crossing when water is above the knees.
- Do not try to swim beyond your personal capacity.
- Learn to swim and teach children to swim.
- Never swim under the influence of drugs and/or alcohol.
- Swim across rip tides.
- Take a surf lifesaver course.
- Use flotation devices.
- Watch children closely near water.
- Wear a helmet during water sports, e.g., kayaking.

Related Chapters

- Diagnosis and Treatment > Environmentally Induced > Cold and/or Water Induced > Hypothermia
- Must Read > Immediate First Aid > Critical First Aid

FROSTBITE

Frostbite is the freezing of the water in the cells. The most commonly affected areas are the earlobes, nose, fingers, and toes.

Frostnip is a very mild form of frostbite. Frostnip does not do any permanent damage to the skin.

Exposure to the cold is the main cause, but things such as constriction, e.g., tight boots, dehydration, exhaustion, prior cold injuries, and vasoconstrictors such as coffee or nicotine are also contributing factors.

Symptoms of Frostbite

There are three levels of severity: superficial, partial, and severe.

Superficial frostbite symptoms include:

- Cold and discomfort.
- Normal perfusion.
- Pink or pale complexion.

Partial-thickness frostbite symptoms include:

- Reduced perfusion.
- Numbness.
- Pallor and softness of skin.

Treatment for Frostnip and Superficial and Partial Frostbite

Note: Thawing tissue and refreezing it will create more damage. Unless a stable environment is more than 24 hours away, it is best to wait.

- Do not drink alcohol or smoke.
- Do not massage or rub the affected area.

- Elevate the extremity.
- Initiate general rewarming of whole body.
- Loosen constrictive clothing.
- Maintain food and water intake.
- Rewarm the affected body part with heat packs, skin-to-skin contact (do not rub or massage), warm water, etc.
- When rewarming, be careful not to burn the patient as he/she may not feel it.
- Analgesics before rewarming

Symptoms of Full-Thickness Frostbite

- Numbness
- Pale and hard body part
- Possible ice crystals
- Perfusion absent

Note: If the skin turns black, it has died from a loss of circulation, a condition known as gangrene. Amputation is usually necessary.

Treatment for Full-Thickness Frostbite

- Immersion of frozen area in 37 to 39 °C (98 to 102 °F) water
- Dry dressings. Separate digits when bandaging.
- Analgesics before rewarming
- NSAIDs for circulation

Prevention of Frostbite

- Avoid alcohol and tobacco.
- Avoid handling cold liquids and metals, especially fuel.
- Avoid wind, especially at high altitudes.
- Do not over-wash as it can wash away natural protective oils.

- Keep covered and warm.
- Keep well rested.
- Maintain hydration and nutrition.
- Minimize cold exposure.

Related Chapters

- Must Read > Immediate First Aid > Critical First Aid > Circulation > Perfusion
- Diagnosis and Treatments > Musculoskeletal System > Amputations

HYPOTHERMIA

Hypothermia occurs when cold temperatures overwhelm the body's ability to produce and retain heat.

Symptoms of Hypothermia

Hypothermia can be mild or severe, and it progresses through very definite symptoms, i.e., when untreated, mild hypothermia will progress into severe hypothermia.

Symptoms of mild hypothermia:

- Body temperature between 35.5 °C (96 °F) and 32 °C (90 °F)
- Difficulty speaking
- Intense shivering
- Irritability
- Lethargy
- Loss of fine motor coordination
- Sluggish thinking
- Violent shivering
- Withdrawal

Symptoms of severe hypothermia:

- Body temperature below 32 °C (90 °F)
- Blue, puffy skin
- Coma
- Depressed vital signs (e.g., pulse, respiratory rate, blood pressure)
- Jerky movements
- Muscular rigidity, i.e., no more shivering
- Respiratory and cardiac failure

Treatment for Hypothermia

- The treatment, whether mild or severe, is basically the same. The earlier you treat hypothermia the better.
- Cover the top of the head.
- Do not rub or massage extremities (in case of frostbite).
- Apply heat packs on armpits, chest, groin, and neck.
- Insulate from below and above, starting from the ground up.
- Increase heat production, i.e., exercise.

Note: Only exercise after sufficient food and fluid has been administrated and when mental status has improved.

- Remove causes, e.g., block the wind, remove wet layers, etc.
- Provide warm, non-alcoholic, and non-caffeinated liquid (only if patient is capable).
- Immersion heating (e.g., a warm bath) only if in a controlled environment; the possibility of after-chill may make it worse.

Rewarming a patient with skin-to-skin contact inside of a sleeping bag (or similar) is a survival technique but may cause the body temperatures of all involved to drop.

Prevention of Hypothermia

- Acclimatize to cold weather.
- Avoid alcohol and other recreational substance use.
- Dress appropriately.

Hypothermia Packaging

Hypothermia packaging is useful when you need to transport the patient, and even if you do not it is a great way to keep the patient warm.

- Ensure the patient is dry.
- Keep patient horizontal.
- Stabilize any injuries, including covering any open wounds.
- Sandwich the patient between layers of insulation and waterproof layers.

Suggested hypothermia packaging:

- The face should be partially covered, but allow for breathing, monitoring, etc.
- Place a large plastic sheet on the ground.
- Next, place an insulated sleeping pad on top of the sheet.
- On the pad, place a sleeping bag (or blankets or whatever you have).
- The patient goes on top of this, along with heating bottles, IVs, etc.
- Fold tops and bottom over the patient, then fold the corners over.
- Fold the sides over, keeping wrinkles to a minimum.
- Strap in place.

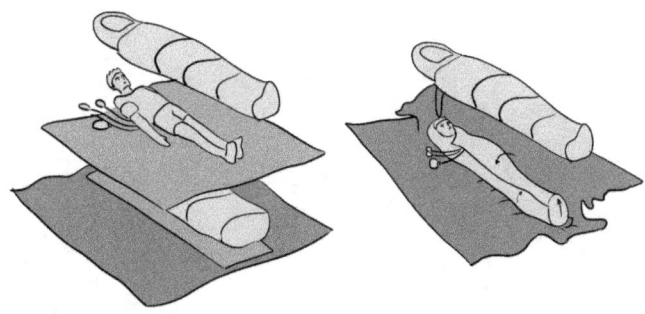

SALTWATER SORES

When a break in the skin is continuously exposed to salt water, saltwater sores may appear. They may also appear where clothing is tight, e.g., at the wrists or ankles.

If in a survival-at-sea situation, prevent sores by not dampening yourself too much with salt water, and change positions frequently.

Symptoms of Saltwater Sores

- Scabs
- Pus

Treatment for Saltwater Sores

- Do not open or squeeze sores.
- Flush with fresh water.
- Keep dry.
- Use antiseptic.

TRENCH FOOT

Trench foot (immersion foot) occurs when the skin is immersed in water (or similar) for an extended period of time. A minor form of this is evident when you have been in a pool and your hands get wrinkled. A more serious case may happen in a survival situation when you have been unable to take off wet shoes for an extended period of time.

Symptoms of Trench Foot

- Red skin that becomes pale and extremely edematous (filled with fluid)

Initial symptoms:

- Decreased perfusion
- Leg cramps
- Numbness
- Pain
- Paresthesia (tingling)

After 2 to 7 days:

- Blisters
- Edema (swelling from fluid)
- Ulceration

After 7 days:

- Stabbing pain

Treatment for Trench Foot

- Avoid use of affected part; if use is unavoidable, at least wear dry, loose-fitting shoes and socks.
- Do not apply creams or ointments.
- Elevate the extremity.
- Keep area dry, warm, and open to air.
- Pat dry (do not rub).

Prevention of Trench Foot

- Keep feet dry and change to a dry pair of socks at least once a day.
- Maintain body core temperature.
- Remain active.
- Remove your shoes when going to bed at night.
- Periodically remove your shoes and socks and rub your feet for 5 to 10 minutes.

Related Chapters

- Must Read > Immediate First Aid > Critical First Aid > Circulation

DIVING INDUCED

There are many things that can wrong when diving, but it is an activity that is usually (and should only be) done under the guidance of a trained professional who should know what to do.

All potential SCUBA divers should seek the advice of a medical practitioner to ensure they are able to participate in the activity, as some conditions are not suitable, e.g., epilepsy, pregnancy, severe asthma, and various lung disorders.

Note: Some of these conditions may occur when flying due to pressure changes.

Do not SCUBA dive if:

- Flying within 12 hours after your last dive.
- Flying within 24 hours of making multiple dives over repeated days or dives that require decompression stops.

ALTERNOBARIC VERTIGO

Alternobaric vertigo usually occurs with ascent and is due to divers' ears not equalizing pressure at the same rate.

It can happen to anyone but is more common in those with a history of eustachian tube dysfunction or middle ear infections.

Symptoms of Alternobaric Vertigo

The telltale symptom is a feeling of vertigo (perception of motion, usually spinning). Other symptoms include:

- Ear pain.
- Feeling of fullness in only one ear.
- Muffled hearing in one ear.
- Nausea.
- Spinning sensation.
- Sounds in one ear, e.g., hissing or ringing.

Treatment for Alternobaric Vertigo

Symptoms usually resolve quickly (typically within minutes). Symptoms that persist for longer than a few hours or are frequently reoccurring may be a sign of something more serious.

If affected during ascent:

- Stop ascending.
- Descend a meter or so and stabilize until sensation passes.
- Do the same if experienced on descent, but ascend a meter or so.

If patient still has vertigo on surfacing:

- Lie down with head elevated 30 degrees.

- Discontinue diving until cleared by a professional.

Prevention of Alternobaric Vertigo

- Ascend and descend slowly.
- Do not dive if sick or congested or have been so recently.
- Do not dive if unusual difficulty clearing ears on descent is experienced.
- Equalize your ears early and often on descent.

Related Chapters

- Diagnosis and Treatment > Head > Ears > Ear Infections > Otitis Media

ARTERIAL GAS EMBOLISM

An arterial gas embolism occurs when air bubbles enter the circulatory system due to ruptured alveoli. It usually occurs immediately after resurfacing and is deadly.

Symptoms of Arterial Gas Embolism

Sudden loss of consciousness upon resurfacing is the major symptom and should be considered an arterial gas embolism until proven otherwise. Other symptoms include:

- Air bubbles in the retinal vessels of the eye.
- Bloody froth from mouth or nose.
- Blurred vision.
- Chest pain.
- Convulsions.
- Disorientation.
- Dizziness.
- Paralysis or weakness.
- Personality change.
- Respiratory arrest.
- Skin marbling.

Treatment for Arterial Gas Embolism

Treat critical systems and other complications as needed, e.g., CPR, hypothermia, etc.

- Get patient to recompression chamber ASAP.
- Hydrate carefully.
- Lie the patient down in a horizontal, neutral position.
- Supply oxygen.
- If traveling in an unpressurized aircraft, fly as low as possible—maximum of 300 m (980 ft) above sea level.

CONTAMINATED BREATHING GAS

Carbon monoxide or oil may be present in the scuba tank.

Symptoms of Contaminated Breathing Gas

Carbon monoxide:

- Dizziness while diving
- Headache
- Mental dullness
- Lethargy
- Nausea

Oil contamination:

- Cough
- Shortness of breath
- Oily taste

Treatment for Contaminated Breathing Gas

- PROP

Related Chapters

- Must Read > Immediate First Aid > Critical First Aid > Breathing

DECOMPRESSION SICKNESS

Decompression sickness (i.e., DCS, diver's disease, the bends, caisson disease) is the formation of bubbles in the body and can affect almost any area of the body, e.g., the brain, heart, joints, and skin.

It usually occurs when a diver resurfaces too fast, and the risk is directly related to the depth of the dive, i.e., the deeper a diver goes, the higher the risk.

Symptoms of Decompression Sickness

Symptoms will occur within 48 hours but are more likely within 6 hours. These include:

- Abdominal pain.
- Back pain.
- Chest pain.
- Extremity heaviness, weakness, or paresthesia.
- Fatigue.
- Joint pain and tenderness, especially in shoulders and elbows.
- Sphincter weakness.

Staggers:

- Possible but not always present
- Deafness
- Ringing in the ears
- Spinning sensation
- Vomiting

The chokes:

- Rare but serious
- Burning pain in chest, especially on inhalation

- Cough
- Cyanosis (blue lips and skin)
- Respiratory problems

Treatment for Decompression Sickness

Treat critical systems and other complications as needed, e.g., CPR, hypothermia.

- Get patient to recompression chamber ASAP.
- Lie the patient down in a horizontal, neutral position.
- Supply oxygen.
- If traveling in an unpressurized aircraft, fly as low as possible—maximum of 300 m (980 ft.) above sea level.

Note: DCS does not only affect scuba divers; it can also occur at high altitude (e.g., in flying and aerospace environments).

INNER EAR BAROTRAUMA

Inner ear barotrauma most commonly occurs when a diver attempts to forcefully equalize his/her ears, which can result in deafness or vestibular disorders (parts of the inner ear and brain that help control balance and eye movements).

Symptoms of Inner Ear Barotrauma

Symptoms may develop immediately or after hours.

- Hearing loss
- Feeling of fullness in the ear
- Tinnitus (ringing in the ears)
- Vertigo (perception of motion, usually spinning)
- Vomiting

Treatment for Inner Ear Barotrauma

- Rest with head elevated approximately 30 degrees.
- Seek advanced medical care.

MASK SQUEEZE

Mask squeeze occurs when the air space in a divers mask is not equalized during descent. It is easily prevented by exhaling periodically into the mask from the nose when descending and anytime suction is felt on the face. Exhaling into the mask after each time you do ear equalization is good practice.

Mask squeeze is not usually dangerous, although severe mask squeeze can be.

Symptoms of Mask Squeeze

- Blood in white of eyes
- Raccoon-like bruises over/around cheeks and eyes

Treatment for Mark Squeeze

- Mask squeeze is self-resolving. The color will probably fade to green or yellow before disappearing.
- Antibiotic drops (Cortisporin) can help in severe cases to prevent infection.

NITROGEN NARCOSIS

Nitrogen narcosis occurs when a diver gets intoxicated by the nitrogen inside the compressed air tank. Severe cases can lead to death.

Most divers experience symptoms of nitrogen narcosis at depths greater than 30 m (100 ft.), but it can occur in as little as 10 m of water. For this reason, it is not recommended to use compressed air deeper than 35 m (120 ft.).

Symptoms of Nitrogen Narcosis

Symptoms progressively worsen with depth.

- Decreased coordination
- Euphoria
- Giddiness
- Light-headedness

Severe symptoms:

- Hallucination (sight and sound)
- Increasingly poor judgment
- Overconfidence
- Slowed reflexes
- Unconsciousness

Treatment for Nitrogen Narcosis

- Ascend and stay in shallower water until symptoms resolve.
- If symptoms do not resolve, there is another cause for the symptoms.

HOT TUB FOLLICULITIS

Hot tub folliculitis (pseudomonas folliculitis) is a skin infection that can occur after being in heated recreational water sources or from wearing a wet suit that has not been washed and dried properly after the previous use.

Symptoms of Hot Tub Folliculitis

Small red itchy or tender bumps usually appear within 48 hours of exposure and usually in areas covered by the bathing suit/wet suit and are accompanied by:

- Earache.
- Headache.
- Mild fever.
- Nausea.
- Sore throat.
- Vomiting.

Treatment for Hot Tub Folliculitis

- Antihistamine.
- Drying lotions, e.g., Calamine.

PULMONARY BAROTRAUMA

Pulmonary barotrauma (pulmonary over-pressurization syndrome) is a lung injury caused by the expansion of gas in the lungs during ascent in scuba divers and during descent in free diving.

It is not related to depth, dive time, or nitrogen absorption; hence, all divers are susceptible. It is fatal.

It can be caused by holding the breath underwater, pre-existing lung conditions, and/or rapid ascent.

Symptoms of Pulmonary Barotrauma

- Chest pain several hours after diving
- Crepitus (grating feeling or sound)
- Hoarse voice

Severe symptoms:

- Bloody sputum
- Decreased respiratory
- Fainting
- Pneumothorax

Treatment for Pulmonary Barotrauma

- Oxygen
- Prepare for and treat pneumothorax if needed.

Related Chapters

- Diagnosis and Treatments > Musculoskeletal System > Pneumothorax

SINUS SQUEEZE

Sinus squeeze (barosinusitis) happens when pressure inside a sinus cavity causes pain. It commonly occurs if a diver has nasal congestion due to the inability to equalize sinus pressure.

Symptoms of Sinus Squeeze

- Pain in and over the affected sinus (main symptom)
- Possible bloody nose

Treatment for Sinus Squeeze

- Avoid diving until recovered
- Warm compress to the face
- Monitor for development of sinusitis and treat if needed.
- Decongestant
- Corticosteroid

Related Chapters

- Diagnosis and Treatments > Head > Nose > Sinusitis

TOOTH SQUEEZE

Tooth squeeze (barodontalgia) mostly occurs during ascent. It is when gas/air gets trapped in either a cavity or filling, which causes pressure resulting in pain.

Symptoms of Tooth Squeeze

- Bleeding around gums
- Broken tooth
- Tooth pain after diving

Note: Pain in the face and upper teeth is probably sinus squeeze.

Treatment for Tooth Squeeze

- Pain will dissipate over time.
- Discontinue diving until recovered.
- Treat symptoms.

Related Chapters

- Diagnosis and Treatments > Environmentally Induced > Cold and/or Water Induced > Diving Induced > Sinus Squeeze

HEAT AND/OR SUN INDUCED

GENERAL PREVENTION OF HEAT-RELATED ILLNESSES

- Avoid drugs (including medical) and alcohol.
- Maintain adequate hydration and nutrition.
- Take the time to acclimatize.

Acclimatizing to Heat

Most heat-related illnesses can be prevented with proper acclimatization, i.e., the body will be able to deal with the heat if introduced to working in it in a controlled manner.

Acclimatize in similar conditions to what you will be in, e.g., if you are going somewhere hot and humid, it is best to acclimatize somewhere hot and humid.

Exercise moderately for 1 to 2 hours a day for 8 to 10 days.

As the days go on, gradually increase intensity and time spent working.

BURNS

A burn is a flesh or skin injury caused by exposure to and/or contact with heat, electricity, chemicals, friction, or radiation.

Symptoms of Burns

The seriousness of burns is often categorized by their degree.

Superficial/first degree:

- Affects only the superficial skin (the epidermis).
- Red, warm, and dry
- Painful to touch
- Discomfort usually diminishes after 24 to 48 hours.

Partial thickness/second degree:

- Affects some underlying layers of the skin.
- Blisters
- Clear or whitish fluid
- Moist
- Swollen

Full thickness/third degree:

- Affects all layers of the skin and possibly even fat and/or muscle.
- May appear charred or white.
- May appear indented.
- May cause shock.

Treatment for Burns

First:

- Remove the heat source.
- If clothing is on fire, roll on the ground or suffocate the flames, e.g., with a blanket.
- If it is a chemical burn or the eyes are involved, flush with copious amounts of water for at least 10 minutes.
- If phosphorous, keep burn immersed in water.

Next:

- Remove watches, jewelry, constrictive clothing, etc.
- Apply cool (not ice cold) water for at least 10 to 15 minutes.

Note: If 30 minutes of cooling has no benefit other than comfort:

- Consider draining large blisters.
- Clean, cover, and monitor.
- Hydrate.
- Wear loose, light clothing, e.g., cotton.
- Full-thickness burns may require a skin graft to heal.
- Apply burn cream.

Alternative Remedies for Burns

There are a number of well-known alternative remedies to help heal and/or soothe first or perhaps even second-degree burns.

Aloe Vera: Split open a leaf and rub the gel directly on the burn every couple of hours.

Black tea: Make yourself a cup of tea and then apply the used teabag topically.

Plantain: Use as a poultice.

Tannin: Use as a compress.

Honey (raw):

- Pour clean honey liberally over and all around the burned area.
- Wrap with plastic wrap and secure with a bandage.
- After 48 hours, check for infection; treat if present, although it is not likely.
- Remove charred or loose flesh; do not force removal if stuck to the wound.
- Pour more honey over the wound and re-cover.
- Repeat process every 2 days. Every time you open the dressing, add more honey. Do not wash off the honey.
- After 7 to 10 days, the wound will begin to granulate. Do not wash. Leave the dressing off for an hour, then apply more honey and re-cover.
- Remove dressing every 2 hours, and leave open for an hour longer each day.
- After 3 weeks of doing this, you can wash the honey off. Do not use anything but clear, running, drinking-quality water.
- Continue to lightly dress.

Vinegar:

- A diluted 50/50 mix of vinegar and water will cool the burn and also help disinfect it.
- Soak material in the mix and apply it to the burn.
- Reapply as needed.
- Vinegar could also be added to a cool bath to soak clothing the patient will wear, etc.

Yoghurt:

- Use full-fat yoghurt.
- Smother the burn in yogurt.
- Wait 15 minutes, then bathe in cool water.
- Could also be used as a compress.

Do not:

- Use lotion, grease, butter, etc.
- Remove embedded, charred material that will cause burned areas to bleed.
- Move or rub the burned part.

Prevention of Burns

The two most common causes of burn injury are sun exposure and cooking accidents.

Prevention of sunburn:

Be sun-safe. Minimize time in the sun, and when you are in the sun, 'slip, slop, slap, and seek':

- **Slip** on a shirt and long clothes in general.
- **Slop** on lots of sunscreen regularly when exposed to the sun (minimum SPF 30).
- **Slap** on a wide-brimmed hat and sunglasses.
- **Seek** out shade and minimize time in the sun.

Prevention of cooking burns:

- Protect yourself while cooking, e.g., hand protection.
- If you need to test whether something is hot, use the back of your hand.

Related Chapters

- Diagnosis and Treatments > Integumentary System > Blisters and Hot Spots
- Must Read > Open Wounds, Skin Infections, and Sepsis > Open Wounds

HEAT EDEMA

Heat edema is the swelling of extremities due to the heat. It may develop in the first few days of being in a hot climate.

Treatment for Heat Edema

- Avoid diuretics, e.g., coffee.
- Elevate the affected limb.
- Swelling will decrease in time.

HEAT EXHAUSTION

Heat exhaustion occurs when fluid loss is greater than fluid intake. It often occurs after strenuous activity in high temperatures.

The patient may also be dehydrated.

Symptoms of Heat Exhaustion

- Chills
- Dizziness
- Elevated respirations, pulse, and temperature
- Headache
- Nausea
- Sweating
- Vomiting

Treatment for Heat Exhaustion

- Rehydration
- Place a moist, cold compress on the armpits, chest, groin, and neck.
- Remove restrictive clothing.
- Rest in a cool environment.

Related Chapters

- Diagnosis and Treatments > Circulatory System > Dehydration and Volume Shock > Dehydration
- Diagnosis and Treatments > Circulatory System > Dehydration and Volume Shock > Rehydration Plan

HEAT RASH

Heat rash (prickly heat) occurs when the sweat ducts become blocked and swell. It is usually found on body areas covered by clothing.

Symptoms of Heat Rash

- Itching
- Red or pink rash-like dots or tiny pimples

Treatment for Heat Rash

- Avoid ointments or other lotions.
- Dry and cool affected site.
- Heat rash will usually dissipate within 10 days.
- Loosen or remove clothing.
- Antihistamine

HEAT STROKE

Heat stroke occurs when the body produces more heat than it can expel. It may or may not be preceded by heat exhaustion. It is life threatening.

Symptoms of Heat Stroke

- Body temperature above 40.5 °C (105 °F)
- Decreased blood pressure
- Altered (depressed) mental state
- Elevated pulse
- Elevated respiration
- Flushed or pale skin
- Seizures
- Sweat may or may not be present.

Treatment for Heat Stroke

- Elevate legs above the heart.
- Rapid cooling (e.g., cold water immersion, saturating and fanning, lying in a stream). Be careful not to overcool.
- Rest
- Rehydration
- Continue to cool until core temperature returns to normal, i.e., 38 to 39 °C (100.4 °F to 102.2 °F); check every 30 minutes.
- Maintain airway, breathing, and circulation.
- Benzodiazepine to treat seizures and shivering

Prevention of Heat Stroke

- Avoid drugs (including medical) and alcohol.
- Maintain adequate hydration and nutrition.

- Take the time to acclimatize.

Related Chapters

- Diagnosis and Treatments > Head > Brain > Seizure
- Diagnosis and Treatments > Circulatory System > Dehydration and Volume Shock > Rehydration Plan
- Must Read > Immediate First Aid > Critical First Aid

HEAT SYNCOPE

Heat syncope is fainting as a result of low blood pressure due to overheating. It usually occurs due to standing in a hot environment for too long or standing up too fast.

Treatment for Heat Syncope

- Cool the patient.
- In case of a fall, perform a full secondary assessment.
- Lay the patient flat and elevate his/her legs 15 to 30 degrees above the heart.
- Provide oral fluids when the patient is alert.
- If recovery does not occur after treatment, assess for more serious heat illnesses, e.g., heatstroke.

Related Chapters

- Diagnosis and Treatments > Environmentally Induced > Heat and/or Sun Induced > Heat Stroke

HYPONATREMIA

Hyponatremia occurs when there is excessive water consumption with inadequate salt replacement, e.g., when someone sweats a lot and drinks water to stay hydrated but does not eat to replace salts.

Symptoms of Hyponatremia

- Decreased mental status
- Dizziness
- Headache
- Muscle cramps
- Nausea
- Loss of coordination
- Tremors
- Vomiting
- Vital signs and core temperature are often normal or only slightly irregular

Treatment for Hyponatremia

- Drink a full-strength sports drink but only if mental status is okay.
- Eat when able.
- If unable to drink, intravenous therapy may be needed.

MISCELLANEOUS ENVIRONMENTAL ILLNESSES

ALLERGIC REACTIONS

An allergic reaction is actually a defense of the body. It is an overreaction of the immune system to an otherwise harmless substance.

Although knowledge of a previous history of allergic reaction can help identify the cause, it is not set in stone. Allergic reactions can happen even without precedent, and previous allergies may go away. Also, the severity of reactions is not always the same. What might cause eye irritation one time may result in anaphylaxis the next.

Almost anything can cause an allergic reaction. It is dependent on the person. Some common examples are animals, dust, foods (usually within 30 minutes), insects (allergic reaction from stings usually occur within 5 minutes), medications (usually within 30 minutes), and plants.

Symptoms of Allergic Reactions

Symptoms are varied. Some common ones are:

- Eye irritation and/or redness. The big difference from an eye infection is the lack of milky discharge.
- Gastrointestinal problems, e.g., diarrhea.
- Hives.
- Rash.
- Sneezing.
- Stuffy nose.
- Swelling.
- Wheezing.

Treatment for Allergic Reactions

- Treat symptoms.
- Clean, dry, and ventilate the area well.
- Remove the cause.

- Monitor for signs of anaphylaxis.
- Antihistamine
- For hives or rashes, make a poultice out of fresh cilantro and apply it topically.

Prevention of Allergic Reactions

- Avoid contact with known irritants.
- Wear long clothing.
- Apply topical creams as barriers.
- Perform post-exposure washes.

Related Chapters

- Must Read > Immediate First Aid > Anaphylaxis

HAY FEVER

Hay fever is a common allergic reaction specifically to something that has been breathed in, e.g., dust, fungi, or pollens.

Symptoms of Hay Fever

- Irritated eyes
- Itchy skin
- Itchy throat
- Nasal congestion
- Red eyes
- Sneezing
- Tearing

Treatment for Hay Fever

- Treat symptoms.
- Clean, dry, and ventilate the area well.
- Remove cause.
- Antihistamine

CARBON MONOXIDE POISONING

Carbon monoxide poisoning usually occurs when too much carbon monoxide accumulates in a confined space. It is produced by appliances that burn fuel or gas, e.g., automobiles, heaters, fireplaces, etc., and also by fire in general, e.g., structure or forest fires.

Breathing in too much carbon monoxide reduces the body's ability to absorb oxygen, which leads to tissue damage, brain damage, and eventually death.

Unfortunately, carbon monoxide is difficult to detect as it is a colorless, odorless, and tasteless gas. People who are intoxicated or sleeping often do not feel the effects before it is too late, meaning they are at greater risk.

Symptoms of Carbon Monoxide Poisoning

- Altered mental state
- Blurred vision
- Dizziness
- Headache
- Lethargy
- Loss of consciousness
- Loss of coordination
- Nausea
- Shortness of breath
- Vomiting

Treatment for Carbon Monoxide Poisoning

- PROP
- Seek advanced medical care.

Related Chapters

- Must Read > Immediate First Aid > Critical First Aid > Breathing

JET LAG

Jet lag (desynchronosis) occurs when your internal clock gets messed up due to crossing time zones too quickly, i.e., when traveling by plane. The problem occurs because your body is not used to the new daylight and darkness patterns.

This means that if you are traveling north/south along the same timeline, jet lag will not occur, no matter how long the flight is. Of course, you may not feel 100% due to a number of reasons, but jet lag just won't be one of them in this case.

For most people, jet lag is only a problem when crossing two or more time zones. The time it takes for the body to adjust is dependent on the person and the number of time zones crossed.

Symptoms of Jet Lag

Fatigue and/or insomnia are the major symptoms. Others may include:

- Anxiety.
- Constipation.
- Diarrhea.
- Irritability.
- Nausea.

Treatment for Jet Lag

Most people can expect their bodies to adjust at a rate of one or two time zones per day. This process can be made faster by helping the body adjust to the new time zone.

- Change your watch to the new time zone and synchronize your routine to this new time zone including eating, exercising, sleeping, using the bathroom, etc.

- If you must nap, only do so for a maximum of one hour.
- Avoid alcohol, caffeine, and other drugs, including sleeping aids.
- Keep hydrated.
- Move about the plane.
- If possible, you can start this process a few days before you take off. In doing so, your body will not have to make as big an adjustment:
- If traveling east, go to bed an hour or two earlier.
- If traveling west, make it an hour or two later.

LIGHTNING

Although rare, getting struck by lightning is not unheard of. Lightning can be present without rain or visible clouds.

People that have previously been struck or nearly struck are more susceptible, and about one out of every ten people that get struck by lightning die.

There are a number of ways lightning can cause injury, including contact with a conductive material that is hit or splashed by lightning, a direct hit, splash (where it first strikes an item and then 'jumps' to the victim), and vicinity (where the strike is close enough to affect the victim).

Signs of Impending Lightning Strike

- Blue halo around objects
- Hair standing on end
- High-pitched or crackling noises

Symptoms of Lightning Strike

A number of injuries may be sustained from a lightning strike. Common ones are:

- Altered mental state.
- Burns.

Treatment for Lightning Strike

Victims of lightning do not stay 'charged,' so rescuers are safe to treat any injuries that have occurred.

- Treat any injuries.

Prevention of Lightning Strike

- Know the weather forecast.
- If you see lightning and then hear thunder before you can count to 30 seconds:
- Seek shelter in a sturdy building (not a tent or 'tin shed') or a metal-topped vehicle (a sturdy building is preferred).
- Close all windows.
- Avoid all windows, open doors, fireplaces, metal structures, etc.
- Stay inside until 30 minutes after the last lightning is seen and/or the last thunder is heard.

Being in a metal-topped vehicle may seem counter-intuitive. Here is the reasoning:

- A soft-top vehicle will not help you since the lighting will go straight through it.
- If lightning strikes the metal-topped vehicle, it will be grounded due to the tires. You will be safe (safer than outside) as long as you are not touching the metal frame while inside the vehicle.

If there is no adequate shelter:

- If in a group, spread out.
- Avoid cave entrances.
- Avoid exposed areas, isolated tall objects, pools of water, anything metal, wet objects, etc.
- Crouch down on the balls of your feet and tuck your head in, i.e., make yourself as small as possible.
- Do not touch the ground with your hands.
- Insulate yourself from the ground, e.g., with a sleeping pad or rope.
- Seek shelter in low ground.

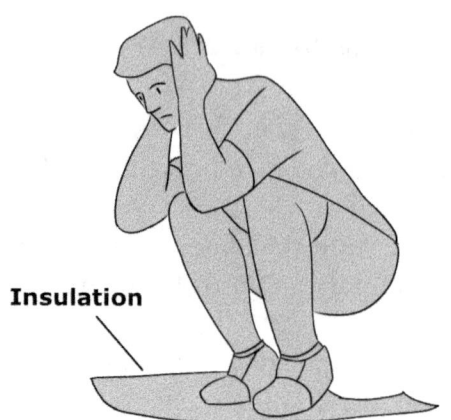

RADIATION SICKNESS

Radiation sickness is probably only likely if exposed to nuclear fallout, and although exposure to such an event may be improbable, it is possible.

Radiation levels are measured in RADs, and small amounts have little effect; in fact, we probably absorb about 0.6 RADs per year in normal settings, e.g., from microwaves.

It is when we are exposed to a big dose in a short period of time that we get sick.

Once Exposed to Radiation

Your number one goal is to decrease your exposure. Do whatever is the best choice for your situation:

- Find shelter.
- Leave the area; the further away you are the better.

Halving Thickness

The effectiveness a material has against radiation in relation to the material's thickness is known as its halving thickness. Denser material has better halving thickness, which means better protection.

One halving thickness will drop the exposure by one half. Doubling it will drop it to one quarter, tripling it will drop it to one eighth, ($1/2 \times 1/2 \times 1/2$), etc.

Here are some halving thicknesses for some common materials:

- Lead: 1 centimeter
- Steel: 2.5 centimeters
- Concrete: 6 centimeters
- Soil (packed): 9 centimeters

- Water: 18 centimeters
- Wood: 30 centimeters

For an illustrative example, if you are in a steel bunker 2.5 cm thick, it will drop your exposure to radiation by one half in comparison to the outside. To drop it by $1/4$, you need a 5-cm-thick bunker.

You can estimate how long you should protect yourself. Radiation levels usually drop by about 1/8th of their level every 24 hours. There are a number of devices available for detecting and measuring radiation.

Symptoms of Radiation Sickness

Different levels of RADs have different effects, and symptoms may arise over time.

At a level of 30 to 70 RADs:

- Full recovery is likely.
- Mild headache or nausea can occur.

At 70 to 150 RADs:

- Full recovery is expected.
- Depressed immune system
- Decreased wound healing
- Mild nausea and vomiting

150 to 300 RADs:

- May cause death.
- Moderate nausea and vomiting
- Fatigue
- Weakened immune system

300 to 500 RADs:

- May cause death.
- Dehydration
- Diarrhea
- Fatigue
- Hair loss (over time)
- Infection
- Moderate nausea and vomiting
- Skin breakdown

Over 500 RADs:

- Death almost certain
- Anorexia
- Bloody diarrhea
- Dehydration
- Fever
- Hair loss
- Infections
- Low blood pressure
- Spontaneous bleeding
- Stomach and intestinal ulcers

Treatment for Radiation Sickness

- Treat symptoms.
- Maintain hydration.
- Maintain food intake.
- Prevent additional exposure.
- Rest.
- Seek advanced medical care.

Prevention of Radiation Sickness

Potassium iodine (KI) will prevent thyroid cancer. Take 130 mg (a standard tablet) 30 minutes to 24 hours prior to radiation exposure, and then once a day during prolonged exposure. Give children half doses.

An alternative to KI is 2% iodine. Put 8 ml on your forearm or stomach 2 to 12 hours prior to exposure. Repeat daily. Only apply 4 ml for children under 70 kg, 2 ml for toddlers, and 1 ml for infants. Cease after 3 days or when radioiodine levels have dropped to safe levels.

Cautions:

- Do not drink iodine; it is poisonous if ingested.
- If allergic to seafood, you will probably be allergic to iodine.
- Use caution if on other medication such as diuretics or lithium.

SMOKE INHALATION

Smoke inhalation is the most common cause of death due to fire and is usually accompanied by burns in the airway.

It can cause asphyxiation (lack of oxygen) and/or chemical irritation.

Symptoms of Smoke Inhalation

- Burns in the mouth, on the face, in the nose, in the pharynx (throat), etc.
- Confusion
- Cough producing black sputum
- Difficulty swallowing
- Drooling
- Headache
- Muffled voice
- Shortness of breath
- Swollen tongue
- Wheezing

Treatment for Smoke Inhalation

- Move patient to clean air (only if safe to do so).
- Treat critical injuries.
- PROP
- Albuterol (common asthmatic medication) may help.

When to seek advanced medical care:

- Difficulty breathing
- Hoarse voice
- Prolonged coughing
- Mental confusion

Related Chapters

- Must Read > Immediate First Aid > Critical First Aid > Breathing

TOXIC PLANTS

There are a wide variety of toxic plants with have a wide range of symptoms, and some can be fatal. Sometimes a part of a plant can be edible while another part is not, e.g., you can eat the flower but not the stem. Others plants be only edible when cooked a certain way. In fact, there are so many plants and so many variables that for a majority of them, no specific treatment exists.

As a rule, do not touch, and especially do not ingest, any plant that you are not 100% sure about.

Treatment for Toxic Plant Contact

- Treat symptoms.
- Use local knowledge.

For skin irritants, e.g., poison oak:

- Thoroughly wash area.
- Use alcohol to neutralize.

If ingested, take the following history:

- Amount and part of plants ingested
- Initial symptoms
- Method of preparation, e.g., drying, cooking, boiling, etc.
- Number of persons who ate the same plant, and their symptoms
- Time between ingestion and onset of symptoms
- Time of ingestion

Do not induce vomiting unless it is a specific treatment, but be prepared for it as a symptom.

Activated charcoal is preferable. If that is unavailable, mix tea and wood charcoal (not briquettes) and add milk of magnesia if available.

Note: Be extra careful of passing on the toxin, e.g., touching your mouth or face after handling or giving rescue breaths.

HEAD

BRAIN

ACUTE STRESS REACTION

Acute stress reaction (ASR) is a stress-related psychological condition that will cause a patient to either panic or faint. Laymen often refer to this as shock, but it is not, though it can occur with shock.

Symptoms of Acute Stress Reaction

- Fainting
- Panic attack

Treatment for Acute Stress Reaction

- Symptoms will subside with time.
- Reassure the patient.
- Treat other problems.

Related Chapters

- Diagnosis and Treatments > Circulatory System > Dehydration and Volume Shock

EPIDURAL HEMATOMA

An epidural hematoma occurs when an artery inside the skull starts to bleed, which results in an expanding blood clot.

Symptoms of an Epidural Hematoma

- Patient wakes from unconsciousness and is normal, only to decline in mental status again, usually within 30 to 60 minutes.
- Unconscious patient with one pupil significantly larger than the other.

Treatment for an Epidural Hematoma

- Seek advanced medical care.

INCREASING INTRACRANIAL PRESSURE

Intracranial pressure (ICP) is pressure in the skull. Increasing ICP to dangerous levels can lead to death.

Causes of Increasing ICP

- HACE
- Infection
- Severe head injury (TBI)
- Stroke

Symptoms of Increasing ICP

Early:

- Change in mental status
- Persistent vomiting
- Severe headache

Late:

- Blown pupils
- Irregular respirations
- Low pulse
- Seizure

Treatment for Increasing ICP

- PROP
- Seek advanced medical care

Related Chapters

- Diagnosis and Treatment > Environmentally Induced > Altitude Induced > HAPE and HACE
- Must Read > Open Wound and Skin Infections
- Diagnosis and Treatment > Head > Traumatic Brain Injury
- Must Read > Immediate First Aid > Critical First Aid > Breathing

INSOMNIA

Insomnia is the inability fall to sleep and/or to stay asleep for as long as you need.

Short-term (acute) insomnia (days or weeks) may be caused by alcohol, caffeine, drugs, nicotine, illness, stress, etc.

Long-term (chronic) insomnia occurs when someone has insomnia three or more nights a week for over a month and may be caused by anxiety, chronic stress, depression, etc.

Symptoms of Insomnia

- Anxiety
- Daytime sleepiness
- Difficulty falling asleep
- Irritability
- Waking during the night and being unable to return to sleep

Treatment for Insomnia

- Treat underlying/contributing cause(s).
- Diphenhydramine: 12 years and older, 25 to 50 mg at bedtime.
- Sleeping pills (caution of dependency)
- Herbal tea: Chamomile tea, ginger, or peppermint after eating
- Salt and sugar: If waking up during the night, sprinkle a little salt and sugar (or salted honey) on the tongue.

Prevention of Insomnia

- Avoid alcohol, caffeine, and nicotine late in the day (at least five hours before).
- Don't eat a heavy meal late in the day, but a light snack before bedtime may help.
- Drink less before going to sleep.
- Exercise regularly but not right before bedtime (at least two hours before).
- Follow a routine to help you relax before sleep, e.g., read a book, listen to music, take a bath, etc.
- Have a comfortable sleeping area (consider noise, temperature, lighting, etc.).
- Have sex or masturbate before sleeping.
- Maintain a consistent sleeping schedule, i.e., wake up and sleep at the same times every day.
- Only use your bed for sleep and sex.

MENINGITIS

Meningitis is an infection of the spinal cord and brain lining, and although rare, it can be fatal in some cases (bacterial meningitis). It is completely different from influenza, but the symptoms are almost exactly the same, which is why it is so dangerous.

Symptoms of Meningitis

The telltale signs of meningitis that differentiate it from influenza are stiffness of the neck and back and the lack of cough or a runny nose. Other symptoms are:

- Fever.
- Headache.
- Intolerance to light.
- High fever.
- Nausea.
- Rapid decline.
- Vomiting.

Treatment for Meningitis

- If you suspect meningitis, seek advanced medical care ASAP.
- Antibiotics: Ampicillin, metronidazole, sulfamethoxazole/trimethoprim

Related Chapters

- Diagnosis and Treatment > Respiratory System > Cold and Flu

SEIZURE

Seizures occur when there are changes in the brain's electrical activity with symptoms ranging from merely staring off into space to violent shaking. The underlying causes are numerous. Basically, anything that affects the body may also disturb the brain and cause a seizure.

Extremely long seizures can lead to coma or death.

Types of Seizures

- **Non-epileptic seizures:** These are typically a result of a head injury or an underlying illness. When the cause is treated, the seizures go away.
- **Partial seizures:** These only affect one side of the body.
- **Generalized seizures:** These affect both sides of the body.
- **Petit mal seizures:** These are not as obvious, and the patient may just be 'absent' for a short time (seconds), e.g., staring off into space.

Symptoms of Seizures

Pre-seizure:

- Altered vision
- Anxiousness or fear
- Dizziness
- Sick to the stomach

Symptoms when a seizure is in progress (may be present for up to 15 minutes):

- Blackout followed by confusion

- Clenching teeth
- Drooling or frothing at the mouth
- Falling
- Loss of bladder or bowel control
- Making unusual noises, such as grunting
- Mood changes
- Muscle spasms
- Rapid eye movements
- Strange taste in the mouth

Treatment for Seizures

- Clear the area around the patient.
- Cushion patient's head.
- Place on his/her side.

When to seek advanced medical care:

- Patient remains unconscious.
- Seizures are repeated.
- Seizure is longer than 3 minutes.

After the seizure:

- Evaluate and treat any injuries.
- Treat underlying cause.
- Regardless of the symptoms, all seizures are a cause for concern, and the patient should always be referred to advanced medical care.
- If the seizures are due to epilepsy, the patient will probably know what to do for aftercare.

STROKE

A stroke is damage to the brain caused when the blood supply to the brain is either interrupted or reduced, e.g., by a burst blood vessel, clot, or high blood pressure. This causes brain cells to die.

Depending on the part of the brain of which the circulation is comprised, the functions of that part of the brain will be affected, e.g., speech, sight, and/or comprehension.

Preventative measures mainly revolve around being healthy in general, e.g., exercise and nutrition.

Symptoms of Stroke

- Altered consciousness
- Confusion
- Dizziness
- Headache
- Lack of coordination
- Loss of vision in one or both eyes
- Paralysis or weakness on one side of the body and/or face
- Slurred speech (or total inability)
- Sudden severe headache
- Trouble with speaking, understanding, etc.
- Vomiting

Treatment for Stroke

The first few days will show the most improvement, if any.

- Seek advanced medical care.
- Bed rest
- Elevate head and torso 30 to 40 degrees.
- Maintain airway.

- Oxygen
- Blood thinners ONLY if you are certain the stroke was caused by a clot

TRAUMATIC BRAIN INJURY

A head injury is considered a traumatic brain injury (TBI) when it results in amnesia, a change of mental status, and/or a loss of consciousness. Usually there is no permanent damage unless the trauma is repeated, e.g., boxers.

Symptoms of a TBI

- Amnesia (memory loss)
- Change of mental status
- Temporary loss of consciousness

Treatment for a TBI

- If unconsciousness for more than 5 to 10 minutes, treat as increasing **ICP**.
- Perform spinal assessment.
- Rest for at least 12 hours.
- Observe for increasing **ICP**.
- Awaken every 2 to 3 hours if sleeping to ensure no symptoms of increasing **ICP**.

Related Chapters

- Diagnosis and Treatments > Head > Increasing Intracranial Pressure
- Must Read > Secondary Exam > Physical Exam

HEADACHES AND MIGRAINES

Headaches are often just a nuisance, but they are also a common symptom of other medical conditions.

Alternative Remedies for Headaches in General

- Place ice pack where the headache is.
- Massage back of neck.
- Massage where the headache is.
- Lie down in a dark, quiet room.
- Sleep.

DEHYDRATION HEADACHE

Dehydration is a common cause of headaches.

Symptoms of Dehydration Headaches

- Pain on both sides which worsens when standing up rapidly

Treatment for Dehydration Headaches

- Hydrate.
- Rest.

SINUS HEADACHE

A sinus headache is caused by a sinus infection.

Symptoms of Sinus Headaches

- Constant pain in the front of the face
- Increased pain with head movement
- Often a one-sided headache

Treatment for Sinus Headaches

- Treat the sinus infection.

Related Chapters

- Diagnosis and Treatment > Head > Nose > Sinusitis

TENSION HEADACHE

This is the most common type of headache and is due to muscle spasms of the neck and head. It can be short-lived (e.g., 20 minutes), or it may last up to a week.

Many things can cause a tension headache, including:

- Anxiety.
- Depression.
- Head injury.
- Head or neck in an abnormal position for a period of time.
- Lack of sleep.
- Poor posture.
- Stress.
- Teeth grinding.

Symptoms of Tension Headache

- Headache on both sides of the head and/or the back of the head and neck
- Sensation of pressure or tightening

Treatment for Tension Headache

- Massage the back of the neck and temples.
- Analgesics

Prevention of Tension Headache

- Identify and avoid the triggers

MIGRAINES

Migraines are recurrent moderate-to-severe headaches, the exact cause of which is uncertain.

Symptoms of Migraines

- Affected vision, e.g., blurring, light sensitivity
- Nausea
- Pain behind the eye (usually one-sided)
- Sensitivity to light, noise, or odors
- Vomiting

Treatment for Migraines

- Bed rest in the dark
- Caffeine
- Sumatriptan, e.g., Imitrex
- Ice where it hurts most and on the back of the neck.
- Keep body and head warm, e.g., hot bath, hot water bottle on feet.

EARS

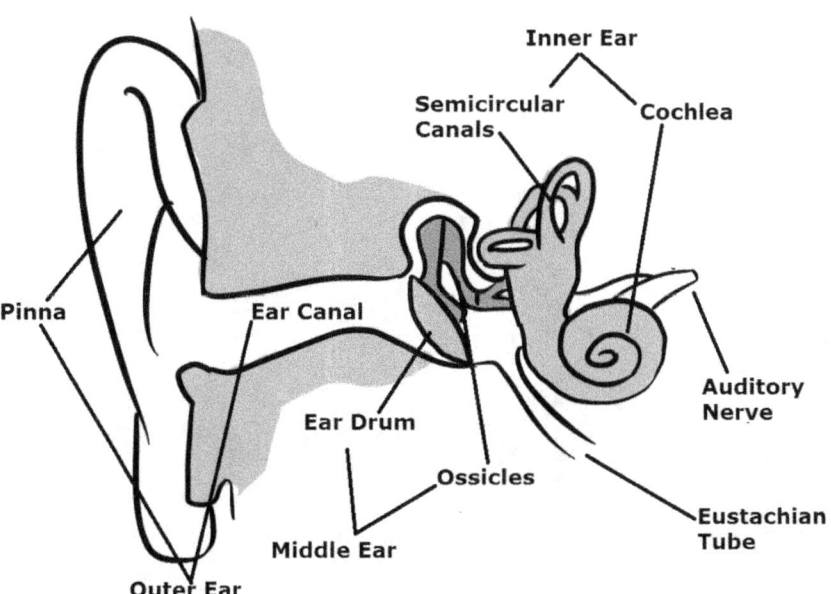

EXTERNAL OTITIS

External otitis (swimmer's ear) is an infection of the outer ear canal. It's most common in children under the age of 15 and usually occurs after long periods of contact with water. It is not contagious.

Another cause is scratching the ear canal, e.g., when trying to clean the ears.

Sometimes the pus from otitis media (middle ear infection) can drain into the canal and cause external otitis.

Symptoms of External Otitis

- Decreased hearing
- Earache
- Itching
- Pain which increases when ear is pulled
- Red, swollen canal
- Tinnitus (ringing in the ears)
- Thick drainage from the ear canal

Treatment for External Otitis

- Keep ear dry if possible.
- Warm compress to soothe the ear
- Antibiotic ear drops, e.g., Cortisporin: 2 to 3 drops in the ear 4 times a day for 7 to 10 days
- Antibiotic, oral for severe cases: Trimethoprim/sulfamethoxazole
- NSAIDs

Prevention of External Otitis

- Dry your ears thoroughly.
- Keep all objects out of your ear canals.
- Use medicated ear drops after swimming.

Related Chapters

- Diagnosis and Treatment > Hear > Ears > Ear Infections > Otitis Media

OTITIS MEDIA

Otitis media (middle ear infection) is the inflammation of the middle ear. It is most common in children and is usually associated with an earache.

Symptoms of Otitis Media

- Dull appearance of eardrum (normally shiny and grayish)
- Earache
- Fever
- Fluid from ear
- Hearing loss
- Holding or pulling the affected ear
- Loss of appetite
- Loss of balance
- Pain, especially when lying down
- Serious symptoms more common in adults

Treatment for Otitis Media

- Will usually self-resolve within 8 days.
- A heat pack may soothe.
- Antibiotics in case of fever, no improvement within 72 hours, pain increase, symptoms of cold, and/or reoccurring infections: Amoxicillin/clavulanate 500 mg every 12 hours for 10 to 14 days or 875 mg every 12 hours for serious cases.
- Antibiotics, other: Amoxicillin, ampicillin, cephalexin, sulfamethoxazole/trimethoprim

Alternative Remedies for Otitis Media

- Clove oil and sesame oil: Mix three drops of pure clove oil in 2 teaspoons of sesame oil, warm it up, and apply in ear.
- Garlic and olive oil: Crush a clove of garlic and mix with a teaspoon of hot olive oil for five minutes. Strain out the garlic. Once cooled, put a few drops at a time into your ear canal.
- Hydrotherapy: This will help drain and soothe the ear. Put a warm compress on the ear for 5 minutes, then a cold one for one minute. Repeat sequence five times, always ending with the cold.

Prevention of Otitis Media

- Dry ears thoroughly.
- Keep all objects out of your ear canals.
- Refrain from bottle/breast feeding with infant lying flat.

EAR WAX

Ear wax is technically known as cerumen. It is normal and protective in healthy ears as it traps dust particles before they can reach the eardrum. Sometimes there can be a lot of build-up of cerumen, which may result in a blocked ear and therefore impaired hearing.

Prevention of this build-up includes regular cleaning of ears, but do not use cotton swabs as you are more likely to just push the wax in further. Also, sticking anything in your ears may lead to a perforated ear drum and/or otitis media.

A much safer alternative is to use a twisted-up wet towel after your daily shower.

Symptoms of Ear Wax Buildup

- Earache
- Impaired hearing
- Itching
- Odor or discharge
- Tinnitus (ringing in the ear)

Treatment for Ear Wax Build-up

- Soften the wax, e.g., with a few drops of warm olive oil.
- Wait ten minutes and then irrigate using a bulb syringe filled with warm water.
- Tilt the ear you are irrigating slightly toward the floor so gravity will direct the water out of your ear.
- Pull the external ear up and back.
- Aim the syringe slightly up and back in the ear canal when squirting.
- You may have to do the olive oil treatment 3 times a day for a few days in stubborn cases.

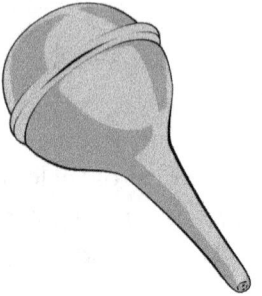

Bulb syringe

Related Chapters

- Diagnosis and Treatments > Head > Ears

FOREIGN BODIES IN THE EAR

Any number of foreign bodies may enter the ear, e.g., dirt, insects, etc. Luckily, the ear canal is very sensitive, so the patient will usually notice if something is in there.

Symptoms of a Foreign Body in the Ear

- Bleeding
- Discomfort
- Impaired hearing
- Nausea or vomiting if it's a live insect
- Sense of fullness in the ear
- If the foreign body is not removed or goes unnoticed, it may lead to an ear infection. Signs of this are swelling or a foul discharge.

Treatment for a Foreign Body in the Ear

- Don't probe or jab.
- Irrigate (bulb syringe or similar) with warm drinking-grade water.
- Do not irrigate in the case of a perforated eardrum.
- Consider extracting object with forceps, though irrigation is usually preferred.

Insects:

- Shine a light to coax them out.
- If that doesn't work, kill the insect with alcohol, 2 % lidocaine, or mineral oil, and then remove as usual.

Related Chapters

- Diagnosis and Treatments > Head > Ears > Ear Infections > Otitis Media
- Diagnosis and Treatments > Head > Ears > Ear Wax

PERFORATED EARDRUM

A perforated eardrum occurs when the eardrum gets ruptured or punctured. It may be caused by air pressure changes (e.g., flying with a severe cold), ear infection, explosion, loud noises, surgery, or trauma.

Symptoms of a Perforated Eardrum

- Can be seen with an otoscope unless infection blocks vision.
- Earache
- Hearing loss
- Mucus discharge
- Tinnitus (ringing in the ears)

Treatment for a Perforated Eardrum

- Usually self-heals within weeks.
- Keep ear clean and dry while healing, e.g., use cotton balls in ear while showering, no swimming.
- Treat infection if needed.

Related Chapters

- Diagnosis and Treatments > Head > Ears > Ear Infections > Otitis Media

EYES

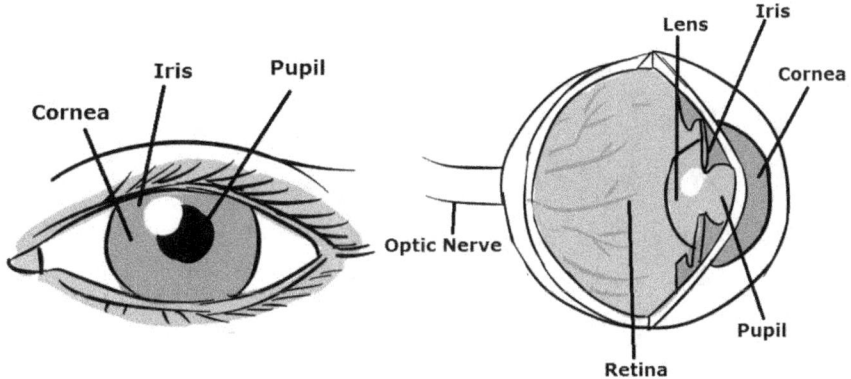

EYE PATCHING

Many treatments of the eye call for patching of the eye. It can offer comfort and may even speed the healing process.

A patch may cause more problems for contact lens users.

- Only patch an eye tightly enough to keep the eyelid shut.
- Fold a gauze square or eye patch in half and place it over the closed eyelid.
- If available, place another patch (unfolded) over the first one and tape completely over the patch from the forehead to the cheekbone.
- If a second patch is not available, just tape the first folded one.
- Inspect and re-patch every 24 hours if needed, using a clean patch every time.

Do your best to not use the eye.

Note: Reading will use both eyes even if one is patched.

When Not to Use an Eye Patch

- Infection is present, e.g., conjunctivitis, corneal ulcer.
- Injury was caused by or contaminated with organic matter.
- Injury is a penetrating injury; instead, use a donut bandage or protective cup to avoid exerting pressure on the eye.

FOREIGN BODIES IN THE EYE

A foreign object is the most likely cause of eye irritation or pain.

Symptoms of a Foreign Body in the Eye

- Irritation
- Pain
- Redness
- Tearing

Treatment for a Foreign Body in the Eye

- Locate the foreign body by examining the corners of the eye and under the eyelids; a moist cotton swab (e.g., Q-tip) can be used to lift and invert the eyelid.
- Irrigate with drinking-quality water (preferably disinfected) from the inside to the outside corner of the eye.
- If the foreign body is not removed by irrigation, dab object off the eye with moist gauze.
- If foreign body is still not removed, patch the eye for 24 hours and then reattempt removal as previously explained.
- After removal, check for corneal abrasion.
- A cool compress can soothe.
- Antibiotic, topical (e.g., erythromycin): Apply to inner surface of lid before patching.

Related Chapters

- Diagnosis and Treatments > Head > Eyes > Corneal Abrasion

CORNEAL ABRASION

A corneal abrasion is a scratch to the cornea.

People that wear contact lenses or have recently had a foreign body in the eye are at higher risk.

Symptoms of Corneal Abrasion

- Grain of sand feeling in the eye
- Irritation
- Redness
- Tearing

Treatment for Corneal Abrasion

- Healing should take a few days depending on the size of the abrasion.
- Remove foreign body if present.
- Irrigate.
- Patch for 24 hours if it makes it feel better.
- If not patched, a cool compress can be applied.
- If it does not heal within four days or gets larger or more painful, seek advanced medical care.
- Antibiotic, topical (e.g., erythromycin): Apply to inner surface of lid before patching.

Related Chapters

- Diagnosis and Treatments > Head > Eyes > Foreign Bodies in the Eye
- Diagnosis and Treatments > Head > Eyes > Eye Patching

ACUTE ANGLE-CLOSURE GLAUCOMA

Acute angle-closure glaucoma (AACG) is caused by a sudden rise of pressure inside your eye, i.e., intraocular pressure. If not treated quickly, it may lead to permanent blindness.

AACG may occur when the pupil is more dilated, e.g., watching television in dim light, excitement, stress.

Some medications may also trigger AACG, e.g., chlorphenamine, cimetidine, eye drops that dilate the pupil, general anesthetic, ipratropium (asthma medication), phenothiazines, ranitidine, SSRI (antidepressant), topiramate, or tricyclic (antidepressant).

Farsighted individuals are more at risk.

Symptoms of Acute Angle-Closure Glaucoma

- Ache around eye
- Blurred or reduced vision
- Dilation of pupil
- Eye feels hard to the touch
- Haloes around eyes
- Headache
- Nausea
- Redness
- Severe pain (sudden)
- Vomiting

Treatment for Acute Angle-Closure Glaucoma

- Seek advanced medical care ASAP.
- Do not cover.
- Adopt a lying-up (supine) position as long as possible.
- Anti-nausea

CONJUNCTIVITIS

Conjunctivitis (pink eye) is a highly contagious eye infection. It is most common in children.

Symptoms of Conjunctivitis

- Eyes 'glued' shut
- Itching
- Photosensitivity (sensitivity to light)
- Pus and/or milky drainage
- Redness

Treatment for Conjunctivitis

- Do not patch.
- Antibiotic, topical (e.g., erythromycin): Apply to inner surface of lid.

Tea eyewashes:

- Chamomile tea (strong)
- Baking soda (half a teaspoon in a cup of water)
- Honey tea (one tablespoon of honey dissolved in a cup of hot water)

Note: Let teas cool before use.

Any of the above eyewashes can also be used as a compress. Apply for 10 minutes every couple of hours.

Prevention of Conjunctivitis

- Change contacts often.
- Don't share eye drops, make-up, etc.
- Keep contacts clean, e.g., don't put them in your mouth.
- Wash hands regularly.

CORNEAL EROSION

As the eyelid opens, a small part of the corneal epithelium (the 'shield' for the cornea) may be torn. It is more common if there is a history of corneal abrasion, and it often happens when first opening the eyes after sleeping.

Symptoms of Corneal Erosion

- Pain
- Photophobia (light sensitivity)

Treatment for Corneal Erosion

- Patch for twelve hours. Re-patch if needed.
- Antibiotic, topical (e.g., erythromycin): Apply to inner surface of lid before patching.
- Lubricant eye drops (e.g., Artificial Tears) every several hours

Related Chapters

- Diagnosis and Treatments > Head > Eyes > Corneal Abrasion
- Diagnosis and Treatments > Head > Eyes > Eye Patching

CORNEAL ULCER

A corneal ulcer is most commonly due to an infection and usually occurs after an injury and/or the use of soft contact lenses.

People who get a lot of cold sores often develop corneal ulcers.

Symptoms of Corneal Ulcers

- Pain
- Photosensitivity (sensitivity to light)
- Redness
- White or gray spot
- May have discharge

Treatment for Corneal Ulcers

- Do not patch.
- Do not wear contact lenses.
- Seek advanced medical care.
- Antibiotic eye drops, preferably gatifloxacin ophthalmic
- Cycloplegic, e.g., atropine, cyclopentolate, etc.

Related Chapters

- Diagnosis and Treatments > Head, Mouth, and Teeth > Cold Sores

DISPLACED CONTACT LENS

Contact lenses can often become displaced. They will not go behind the eye.

Symptoms of a Displaced Contact Lens

- Blurred vision
- Sensation of foreign body in the eye

Treatment for a Displaced Contact Lens

- Ensure the contact lens is still in the eye as it may have fallen out completely.
- Attempt to feel the lens through the eyelid; applying artificial tears may help.
- If you can see the lens, gently slide it back with a finger, and then remove it normally.
- If that is not successful, ask the patient to look down as far as possible as you may then see it.
- The use of a magnifying lens and light may help in finding it.
- Several minutes of gentle massaging over the closed upper lid may cause the contact lens to emerge.
- If that fails, use upward finger pressure to lift the upper lid from the eye and sweep with a moist cotton swab.
- As a final option, fluorescein (a special type of dye) can be used to find it.

GIANT CELL ARTERITIS

Giant cell arteritis (temporal arteritis, cranial arteritis) is a swelling of the lining of the arteries, generally in the head.

Symptoms of Giant Cell Arteritis

- The main symptom is vision loss, which usually affects one eye first. The second eye can be affected within hours or days.
- Fever (low-grade)
- Headache
- Jaw pain
- Ringing in ears
- Stroke (not common)
- Vision loss (rapid and painless)

Treatment for Giant Cell Arteritis

- Immediate pharmaceutical treatment is needed to prevent blindness.
- Seek advanced medical care ASAP for further treatment.
- Treatment should show improvement within a couple of days.
- Corticosteroid, high dose, e.g., prednisone: 100 mg/day.

HYPHEMA

Hyphema is blood in the front of the eye (anterior chamber). It is most likely the result of a blunt injury to the eye and is usually not dangerous unless there is a loss of vision.

It is usually due to some kind of blunt trauma to the eye, but very forceful coughing or sneezing may also cause it.

Symptoms of Hyphema

- Blood in the eye either as a red tinge or a pool
- Decreased vision and eye pain

Treatment for Hyphema

- Hyphema will resolve itself after a while.
- Sit upright and rest.
- Apply a cool compress.
- Keep the head elevated.
- Treat any abrasions.
- Do not patch.
- No NSAIDs
- Cycloplegic, e.g., atropine, cyclopentolate

IMPALING OBJECT IN THE EYE

This is obviously a very serious injury, and loss of vision in the affected eye is possible, especially in a survival situation.

Treatment for an Impaling Object in the Eye

- Stabilize the object.
- Patch both eyes.
- Seek advanced medical care.

If In a survival situation, your options are limited. If no advanced medical care is available:

- If the object is not protruding from the eye, it may be possible to let the wound heal over the object, but that will also increase the chance of infection.
- Removal of the object is the other option.
- A strong magnet may be helpful to remove metal splinters.
- Colloidal silver (taken orally) as well as an eye wash
- If infection starts, surgery must be considered.
- The entire eyeball may have to be removed, which is a very high-risk procedure.

Related Chapters

- Diagnosis and Treatments > Head > Eyes > Eye Patching

SOLAR/ULTRAVIOLET KERATITIS

Solar/ultraviolet keratitis (snow blindness) is a burn to the cornea resulting from intense exposure to UV light. It can occur within one hour, although symptoms may not show for up to 12 hours.

Symptoms of Solar/Ultraviolet Keratitis

- Delayed onset of severe eye pain
- Impaired vision
- Gritty, burning sensation
- Photosensitivity (sensitivity to light)
- Swelling of the eyelid
- Tearing

Treatment for Solar/Ultraviolet Keratitis

- Avoid the sun.
- Remove contact lenses (if applicable).
- Patch.
- Check and replace patch every 12 hours until healed, which is usually within 24 hours. If both eyes are affected and sight is needed, patch the eye that is more severely affected.
- Cold compress can relieve pain.
- Rest.
- Antibiotic, topical (e.g., erythromycin): Apply to inner surface of lid before patching.
- Anesthetic, topical; use only once (to decrease pain during examination).
- NSAIDs

Prevention of Solar/Ultraviolet Keratitis

- Protect eyes from glare, i.e., sunglasses, preferably with side shields.
- Improvised eye protection can be made by cutting slits in a piece of cardboard, duct tape, fabric, etc.

Related Chapters

- Diagnosis and Treatments > Head > Eyes > Eye Patching

STYE

A stye is like a pimple which forms on either the inside or outside of an eyelid. It is due to an infected oil gland, and the main cause is poor hygiene.

Symptoms of a Stye

- Discomfort or pain
- Redness
- Swelling

Treatment for a Stye

Styes may last up to two weeks but can dissipate much faster if treated properly.

- Allow stye to pop on its own.
- Very warm moist compresses for 15 minutes, 4 times daily.
- Close eye while applying compress.
- Antibiotic, topical, e.g., erythromycin (apply to inner surface of lid before patching)

Eyewashes:

- Strong chamomile tea
- Baking soda: 1 teaspoon in 2 cups of cool water
- Honey tea: 1 tablespoon of honey dissolved in a cup of hot water.

Note: Let teas cool before use.

Any of the above eyewashes can also be used as a compress. Apply for ten minutes every couple of hours.

MOUTH AND TEETH

Most issues with the teeth are not easily self-treated and therefore should not be.

When there is no dentist, e.g., in a survival situation, extraction of the problematic tooth will solve most dental emergencies.

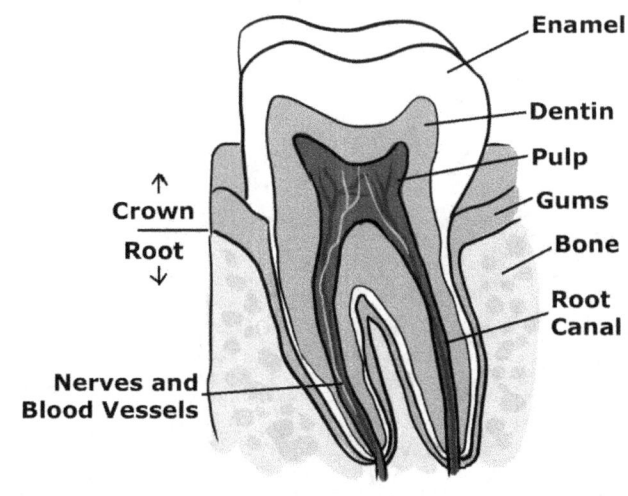

- **Crown:** Above the gum line
- **Root:** Below the crown
- **Alveolus:** Where the tooth sits
- **Ligaments:** What holds the tooth to the alveolus
- **Enamel:** The outside of the tooth, i.e., the white surface that you see
- **Dentin:** Underneath the enamel and surrounding the pulp
- **Pulp:** All the blood vessels, nerves, etc., that are in the middle of the tooth

For Any Dental Procedure

- Wear gloves, mask, eye protection, etc.
- Try to keep the area around the tooth as dry as possible.
- Use cotton balls or rolled gauze around the tooth to help control bleeding.

Related Chapters

- Diagnosis and Treatments > Head > Mouth and Teeth > Dental Extraction

TOOTHACHE

The common toothache (pulpitis) is mainly caused by a bacterial infection, which is a cause of tooth decay. It is an inflammation of the dental pulp tissue.

Symptoms of a Toothache

- Increased sensitivity to hot/cold stimuli
- Throbbing pain radiating to the eye or ear region

Treatment for a Toothache

- Go to a dentist.
- Clove oil applied topically will ease the pain.

If no dentist is available

- Be sure to identify the bad tooth correctly.
- A dental mirror and pick will be useful.
- Look for obvious cavities, abscesses, trauma, etc.
- If nothing obvious is present, use hot/cold stimuli to further investigate.
- Touch the teeth where there is the problem with something cold. A bad tooth is very sensitive to cold.
- Touch this same tooth with something hot.
- If there is pain there, it may need to be extracted.
- If there is no pain to heat, it can be repaired.
- Remove decay and fill.
- If there is no sensitivity to hot or cold but pain to the slightest touch, there is root nerve damage and extraction is needed.
- In a survival situation, the appropriate treatment for a diseased tooth is extraction; the sooner the better.

- NSAIDs

Related Chapters

- Diagnosis and Treatments > Head > Mouth and Teeth > Dental Extraction

EXTRACTION

Extracting a tooth is extremely difficult, especially for an untrained person, and even more so in a survival situation where you may not have access to the proper tools. On the other hand, extraction will fix almost all otherwise non-treatable dental issues. This is good to know if you find yourself in a survival-type situation in which there isn't a dentist.

The procedure will cause lots of pain, so analgesic is advised.

Tools Needed for Field Dental Extraction

- Analgesic
- Elevator
- Extraction forceps
- Gauze

Improvise if the correct tools are not available.

Elevator

Extraction Forceps

Procedure for Field Dental Extraction

Position yourself correctly:

- If you are right handed, stand to the right of the patient, and if you are a left-hander, stand to the left.
- If working on the upper teeth, the patient's mouth is best positioned at your elbow height; have the patient lie head-down at a 60-degree angle to the floor.
- If working on the lower teeth, the patient's mouth is best positioned lower than your elbow, and the patient sits upright.

Most people prefer to be in front of the patient except for the lower molars where you might be better off behind.

Numb the tooth if possible. Clove oil contains eugenol which is well known for being a dental analgesic. Use a high concentration, but be careful as it can burn the mouth, i.e., only apply it to the teeth.

Loosen the tooth. Using a dental elevator or similar (see picture above), apply light pressure between the tooth and gum on all sides to sever the ligaments and get to the root area. It will bleed.

Remove the tooth. If the tooth does not come out after severing the ligaments, use the extraction forceps (or similar) and grip the tooth as far down the root as possible.

Front teeth have one root. Pull them straight out, following the line of the tooth, i.e., directly down or up depending on whether they are upper or lower teeth.

For other teeth, which have more than one root, use a rocking motion to help loosen it as you pull it out. Once loose, extract the tooth away from the tongue.

Commonly, the tooth will break. Use an elevator to push the remainder out.

Put gauze on the bleeding socket. The patient must bite down on it to keep it in place. Heavy bleeding may require stitches.

After-Care of a Tooth Extraction

- Cold packs for first 48 hours to reduce swelling.
- Warm compresses beyond 48 hours to reduce stiffness.
- Do not smoke, spit, use straws, or do anything that may affect the clot.
- No blood thinners, e.g., aspirin, alcohol.
- Only consume cool liquids and soft foods for 72 hours.
- Monitor for dry socket.
- NSAIDs (ibuprofen, because aspirin thins the blood too much)

Related Chapters

- Diagnosis and Treatments > Head > Mouth and Teeth > Dry Socket

AVULSION

Avulsion occurs when the tooth is completely knocked out by some kind of trauma.

Treatment for Avulsion

If you can find and re-implant the tooth within 30 minutes, attempt to do so.

- Avoid touching the roots, i.e., pick it up by the crown.
- Irrigate with saline solution or milk (do not scrub).
- Place in preservation solution if available; if unavailable, place in milk, saline, or saliva rather than plain water.
- Thoroughly empty and irrigate the socket.
- Put the tooth back into the socket with slow, steady pressure.
- Cover it with gauze and have the patient bite down to keep it in place.
- Splint it with soft wax to the neighboring teeth. Candle wax will work if there's nothing else.
- Put the patient on a liquid diet.
- Monitor for dry socket.

Note: Do not replace children's primary (non-adult) teeth.

Related Chapters

- Diagnosis and Treatments > Head > Mouth and Teeth > Dry Socket

DRY SOCKET

Dry socket (alveolar osteitis) occurs in the socket bed after a tooth has been removed. It is due to the absence of a blood clot. It usually results in increased pain and a longer healing time after tooth avulsion or extraction.

Symptoms of Dry Socket

- Clot is gone
- Foul odor in breath
- Bad taste in mouth
- Pain in socket

Treatment for Dry Socket

- Irrigate and redress
- Medicated dressing until pain subsides

Prevention of Dry Socket

- Critical after an avulsion or extraction
- Avoid hot fluids for 48 hours.
- Don't smoke.
- Don't drink through a straw.
- Don't spit forcefully.
- Take recommended medications.

APHTHOUS ULCERS

Aphthous ulcers are non-infectious sores that appear in the mouth. They are usually painful.

The cause is unknown, but they are more common in women than in men. Some medications may trigger them, e.g., nicotine gum.

Patients usually have a history of similar ulcerations.

Symptoms of Aphthous Ulcers

- Burning in the mouth a day or so before an ulcer appears
- Lesion(s) (painful with a red halo)

Treatment for Aphthous Ulcers

The lesions usually dissipate within 10 to 14 days, but some things can be done to speed up the process and/or reduce pain.

- Avoid spicy, salty, and acidic foods and drinks.
- Brush with a soft toothbrush.
- Drink through a straw (not hot liquids).
- Chlorhexidine mouthwash
- Steroid lozenges

BROKEN OR CHIPPED TOOTH

A broken or chipped tooth occurs when a fragment of the tooth breaks off. It may be due to biting down on something hard, trauma, etc.

The sooner it is treated, the more likely the tooth can be fixed.

Symptoms of a Broken or Chipped Tooth

- Pain when exposed to saliva, air, or hot or cold stimuli (food or beverages)
- Visible missing fragments of the tooth

Treatment for a Broken or Chipped Tooth

- Save the pieces of the broken tooth.
- Rinse pieces and wrap in moist fabric.
- Rinse mouth with warm salt water.
- Apply gauze to stop any bleeding; cold water will help also.
- Cover sharp edges with wax or sugarless gum.
- Ice the area.
- Get to a dentist ASAP.
- If no dentist is available, extraction may be needed.

Related Chapters

- Diagnosis and Treatments > Head > Mouth and Teeth > Dental Extraction

COLD SORES

Cold sores (herpes labialis, fever blisters) are the result of an infection that manifests on the lip. They may be caused by dehydration, local skin trauma, menstruation, stress, etc.

They are infectious, so avoid touching the sores, wash hands frequently, and don't share oral items, e.g., water bottles.

Symptoms of Cold Sores

- Early symptom of tingling on the lip
- Small blisters or sores on or around the mouth
- Fever
- Sore throat

Treatment for Cold Sores

- Sores usually dissipate within two to three weeks but are reoccurring.
- Famciclovir and other similar medications are available to speed up healing.
- Garlic: Cut a garlic clove in half and place it directly on the cold sore for 10 minutes several times a day. It may be uncomfortable and/or sting.

CONDENSING OSTEITIS

Condensing osteitis is the inflammation at the root of a tooth, generally as a reaction to an infection.

Symptoms of Condensing Osteitis

- Localized pain
- No obvious swelling
- Sensitive to tapping
- Throbbing

Treatment for Condensing Osteitis

Condensing osteitis is usually self-resolving.

- Soft diet
- Extract as last resort.
- NSAIDs

DENTAL ABSCESS

A dental abscess is a collection of pus around a tooth. It is commonly caused by a bacterial infection which may stem from tooth decay, broken teeth, etc. If untreated, the infection will probably spread to other areas of the body.

In a normal setting, you should go to the dentist. In a survival situation, extraction may be needed.

Symptoms of a Dental Abscess

- Discomfort or pain
- Possible fever
- Sensitivity/pain to touch
- Swelling

Treatment for a Dental Abscess

- Drainage
- Extraction
- Antibiotics alone will not cure a dental infection but can be helpful in reducing symptoms. Use with other treatments, e.g., drainage.
- Antibiotic: Amoxicillin/clavulanate 875 mg two times a day for 7 to 10 days.
- Antibiotic: Amoxicillin

Related Chapters

- Diagnosis and Treatments > Head > Mouth and Teeth > Dental Extraction

FRACTURED TOOTH

A fractured tooth is basically a cracked tooth.

Symptoms of a Fractured Tooth

- May have no symptoms at the start.
- Pain as damage increases to the nerve
- Pain when chewing
- Severe fractures may cause bleeding.

Treatment for a Fractured Tooth

- Stop the bleeding with direct pressure. A moistened teabag works well.
- Cap the exposed area, e.g., candle wax, cavit.
- Reposition the tooth as precisely as possible.
- Splinting is recommended. If no access to specialist equipment, candle wax is better than nothing.
- If the crack extends below the gum line, extract the tooth.

Related Chapters

- Diagnosis and Treatments > Head > Mouth and Teeth > Dental Extraction

GINGIVITIS AND GUM DISEASE

Gingivitis is a bacterial infection of the gums. The exact cause is unknown, but poor oral hygiene is the general cause. If left untreated, gingivitis can progress to periodontitis (gum disease).

Symptoms of Gingivitis

- Bad breath or bad taste in the mouth
- Bleeding gums during and after brushing
- Loose or shifting teeth
- Pockets forming between teeth and gums
- Receding gums
- Red, swollen, or tender gums

Treatment for Gingivitis

Prevention and treatment are the same:

- Brushing
- Flossing
- Mouthwash
- Regular dental check-ups and cleanings
- Antibiotics for serious cases only: Doxycycline 100 mg every 12 hours for 3 days.
- Other antibiotics: Amoxicillin, metronidazole.

LOST FILLING

A lost filling is a previous filling that has fallen out.

Treatment for a Lost Filling

Treatment for a lost filling is the same as for a broken/chipped tooth.

Related Chapters

- Diagnosis and Treatments > Head > Mouth and Teeth > Broken or Chipped Tooth

LUXATION

Luxation in dentistry is basically when a tooth has been pushed out of place, usually from some type of trauma.

Symptoms of Luxation

There are five types of luxation:

- **Concussion:** There is no abnormal displacement or loosening, but the tooth has a reaction to being tapped (percussion).
- **Subluxation (loosening):** A tooth that is knocked loose but is not out of its alveolar socket.
- **Extrusive Luxation**: Partial displacement of the tooth out of its socket; the tooth is usually mobile.
- **Intrusive Luxation:** Displacement of the tooth deeper into the alveolar bone; fracture of the alveolar socket is also usually present.
- **Lateral Luxation:** Eccentric (off-center) displacement of the tooth, usually accompanied by fracture of the alveolar socket. The tooth is usually not mobile, and there is a metallic tone when tapped.

Treatment for Luxation

- Avoid use of affected teeth.
- Splint for severe loosening, e.g., with wax if nothing better is available.
- Soft diet for two weeks
- Extrusive and lateral luxation: Gently and slowly push back in place before splinting.
- Intrusive luxation: Spontaneous re-eruption (self-resolves) or orthodontic extrusion (manually pull it back into position)

MANDIBULAR DISLOCATION

The mandible is the lower part of the jawbone. A dislocation will probably render the patient incapable of closing his/her mouth.

A dislocation of the mandible can be brought on by something as simple as yawning, but if it is caused by trauma, expect a fracture.

Symptoms of Mandibular Dislocation

- Inability to fully open or close the mouth
- Pain

Treatment for Mandibular Dislocation

- Rest your thumbs on the patient's lower molars.
- Move the lower jaw down, then push in, and finally move it up so it 'clicks' back into place.
- Once fixed, the patient should avoid opening the mouth to full extent.

MYOFASCIAL DYSFUNCTION/PAIN

This is immobility or pain in the chewing muscles of the jaw that is usually caused by the grinding of teeth and/or excessive chewing, e.g., eating chewy and/or dried foods.

Symptoms of Myofascial Dysfunction

- Clicking of jaw
- Deviation of the chin to one side on opening
- Headache or earache
- Inability to open the mouth widely
- Limited jaw movement
- Pain in the muscles used for chewing
- Tenderness of jaw muscles

Treatment for Myofascial Dysfunction

- Avoid grinding teeth
- Apply moist heat to jaw
- Eat a soft diet

THRUSH

Thrush is an oral yeast infection that is usually found in the mouth of infants; it sometimes spreads to the nipple tissue of breastfeeding mothers.

Symptoms of Thrush

- Irritation
- White patches in the mouth which may bleed if wiped off

Treatment for Thrush

- Antifungal: Fluconazole once a day for a week.
- Antifungal: Nystatin
- Baking soda solution: 1 tsp in 8 ounces of water applied to nipples.
- White vinegar (distilled): Apply to nipples.
- Yogurt: Apply inside mouth.

TONSILLITIS

Tonsillitis occurs when the tonsils, located at the back of the throat, become infected. It is more common in children than adults.

Symptoms of Tonsillitis

The main symptom is the inflammation of the tonsils. Sometimes swelling results in difficulty of breathing. Other symptoms include:

- Abdominal pain (children).
- Bad breath.
- Blisters or ulcers on the throat.
- Difficulty swallowing.
- Discoloration of tonsils (white or yellow).
- Ear pain.
- Fever.
- Headache.
- Hoarseness.
- Nausea (mainly in children).
- Pain.
- Voice loss.
- Vomiting (mainly in children).

Treatment for Tonsillitis

- Eat soft foods.
- Gargle with warm salt water.
- Lozenges
- Rest
- Warm or very cold fluids to ease throat pain
- Antibiotics in case of a bacterial infection: Amoxicillin, azithromycin
- If viral, it should self-resolve (antibiotics won't work).

NOSE

BROKEN NOSE

A broken nose is a fracture of the nose usually caused by some form of trauma.

Symptoms of a Broken Nose

- Difficulty breathing through the nose
- Pain, especially when pressure is applied
- Possible deformity

Treatment for a Broken Nose

- Consider adjusting obvious deformity back into place, although further damage may be caused.
- Use both hands to straighten the cartilage.
- Consider taping into position.
- Place some ice wrapped in a cloth over the nose for periods of 20 minutes throughout the day; do this for 48 hours.
- Nasal decongestant may help with swelling in the nasal passages.

FOREIGN BODY IN THE NOSE

A foreign body in the nose is something stuck in the nose, e.g., beads, food, rocks, or small parts of toys.

The object may have gotten there voluntarily, e.g., a child sticking something in his or her nose, or by way of trauma.

The object may or may not be in view.

Symptoms of a Foreign Body in the Nose

- Bloody discharge
- Breathing difficulty
- Feeling of something present in the nose
- Foul-smelling discharge
- Pain
- Sensitivity
- Swelling
- Visually seeing something in the nose

Treatment for a Foreign Body in the Nose

- Breathe through the mouth.
- Close the unaffected nostril (press it).
- Blow gently out the nose.

If the above does not work, attempt extraction with tweezers (or similar) but only if you can see the object. If that doesn't work, seek advanced medical care.

Stop extraction if:

- Extreme pain occurs.
- Object moves deeper.

NOSEBLEED

The common nosebleed (epistaxis) is due to a hemorrhage from the nose which may be caused by dry air, excessive picking, hypertension, irritation, trauma, underlying illness, upper respiratory infection, etc.

Treatment for a Nosebleed

- Breathe through the mouth.
- Do not swallow blood; spit it out instead.
- Sit upright with head tipped slightly forward.
- Apply an ice pack to bleeding side of nose.
- Pinch nostrils and push towards the face for 10 to 15 minutes.

If after 15 minutes the nose is still bleeding, repeat the pressure for another 10 to 15 minutes.

If still bleeding, flush with sterile saline, and then gently insert a thin strip of cloth drenched in epinephrine. Do not remove the packing for several hours.

RAW NOSE

A raw nose is a chapped nose, i.e., like chapped lips but on your nose. It most often occurs due to the drying out of the nose from dry air or blowing the nose too much.

Symptoms of a Raw Nose

- Irritation
- Raw inflammation inside nose
- Soreness

Treatment for a Raw Nose

- Avoid hot water on the nose.
- Moisturize the nose, e.g., a damp cloth, face lotion, or petroleum jelly.

Prevention of a Raw Nose

- Keep hydrated.
- Use a humidifier.
- Use special tissues.

SINUSITIS

Sinusitis is a nasal infection.

Symptoms of Sinusitis

- Bad breath
- Cough
- Dental pain
- Facial pain which may increase with head movement
- Facial tenderness
- Fatigue
- Fever
- Headache
- Loss of smell
- Nasal congestion
- Nasal discharge

Treatment for Sinusitis

- Hydration
- Warm facial compresses for relief
- Avoid diphenhydramine.
- Antibiotic: Amoxicillin/clavulanate 500 mg every 12 hours for 10 to 14 days or 875 mg every 12 hours for 10 to 14 days or longer for recurrent and/or more serious cases.
- Antibiotic: Ciprofloxacin 500 mg every 12 hours for 10 days.
- Antibiotics, other: Amoxicillin, ampicillin, azithromycin, levofloxacin, sulfamethoxazole/trimethoprim
- Corticosteroids if severe, e.g., prednisone
- Decongestants and/or NSAIDs
- Nasal vasoconstrictors, e.g., Afrin (do not use for more than five days)

CIRCULATORY SYSTEM

FAINTING

This section covers fainting (syncope) not associated with seizures. A person who faints from a seizure will have jerky movements or will stare into space.

Fainting can be caused by a number of things, e.g., ASR, dehydration, or low blood sugar.

Treatment for Fainting

Unless there is a serious underlying problem, most people will regain alertness shortly.

If the patient feels that he/she is going to faint before it happens, have them sit down and put their head between their knees.

If you see them fainting, gently lower them to the ground, preferably on their back.

Do a critical assessment and treat as needed, e.g., CPR, direct pressure to wounds.

If there is no serious underlying problem:

- Cool the patient if hot.
- Give them fresh air.
- Loosen constrictive clothing.
- Lie patient flat on his/her back and raise their legs 60 cm above their heart/head.
- Slowly sit the patient up when they are ready.
- Have them eat and drink when alert.
- Have them continue to rest until strength returns.
- Assess for other injuries, e.g., concussion from fall.

Related Chapters

- Diagnosis and Treatments > Head > Brain > Seizure
- Must Read > Immediate First Aid > Critical First Aid

INTERNAL BLEEDING

When an artery or vein ruptures, blood will collect inside the body. This is called internal bleeding. Put simply, it is getting a cut inside the body. It can be caused by alcohol and/or drug-induced liver damage, blunt trauma, deceleration trauma, fractures, medication, pregnancy, spontaneous bleeding, etc.

If it occurs in the chest, abdomen, pelvis, retroperitoneum (the space in the abdominal cavity behind the peritoneum), and/or thighs, it can become life threatening.

Symptoms of Internal Bleeding

Symptoms of internal bleeding depend on the part of the body that has suffered damage. Internal bleeding is often accompanied by other medical issues.

- Bruising (localized)
- Bruising on the side indicates abdominal bleeding.
- Black stool indicates bleeding in stomach or small intestine.
- Blood from any orifice (mouth, nose, ears, anus, vagina, or urethra)
- Blood in urine indicates bleeding in the kidney or bladder.
- Decreased mental status indicates bleeding in the brain, e.g., stroke.
- Impaired vision indicates bleeding in the eye.
- Inflammation indicates leaking outside a blood vessel.
- Pain (localized), often at the affected site, e.g., if caused by a fracture
- Pain in chest or that radiates to the shoulder indicates possible bleeding in the diaphragm.
- Volume shock

Treatment for Internal Bleeding

Exact diagnosis and treatment is almost impossible without advanced medical care. The important thing is to notice the possible signs and symptoms so you can seek professional advice earlier rather than later.

- Avoid unnecessary movement of the patient.
- Treat all fractures, in particular an unstable pelvic fracture.
- Treat the cause.

Related Chapters

- Diagnosis and Treatment > Head > Brain > Stroke
- Diagnosis and Treatments > Circulatory System > Dehydration and Volume Shock > Volume Shock

DEHYDRATION AND VOLUME SHOCK

Dehydration occurs when the body loses too much water from things such as diarrhea, sweat, urine, vomiting, etc.

Volume shock, specifically hypovolemic shock, occurs when the body loses too much fluid, i.e., blood and/or water.

Severe dehydration can lead to volume shock, and if volume shock is left untreated, it will lead to death.

Most people (adults) require 2 to 3 liters of fluid replacement each day. This, of course, is highly dependent on many factors, e.g., size, environment, physical exertion, and illness.

DEHYDRATION

Common sense will help prevent dehydration. If you are losing more fluid than normal, replace it. The clearer your urine, the better. If it is dark and/or pungent, drink water.

Symptoms of Dehydration

Mild dehydration occurs when 2% of a person's water content is lost. Symptoms include:

- Anxiety.
- Concentrated urine (darker).
- Decreased work efficiency.
- Loss of appetite.
- Increased rate of pulse and/or respirations.

Moderate dehydration occurs when 4% of a person's water content is lost. As well as the symptoms of mild dehydration, the patient will also experience:

- Decreased blood pressure.
- Dizziness.
- Fatigue.
- Mood swings.
- Nausea.
- Vomiting.

Severe dehydration occurs when 6% of a person's water content is lost. As well as the symptoms of mild and moderate dehydration, the patient will also experience:

- Loss of coordination.
- Decreased skin turgor (when the skin is pulled up for a few seconds and does not return to its original state).

- Incoherence.
- Minimal or no urine output.
- Further decline of vitals.

Treatment for Dehydration

- Treat cause.
- Rehydrate.

Related Chapters

- Diagnosis and Treatments > Circulatory System > Dehydration and Volume Shock > Rehydration Plan

VOLUME SHOCK

Volume shock occurs when there is a major loss of fluid from the body, i.e., blood and/or water loss. It is a deadly complication of a variety of underlying problems, most commonly dehydration or major hemorrhage.

Symptoms of Volume Shock

- Decreased mental status
- Decreased urine output
- Fast breathing
- Pale, cool, and sweaty skin
- Weak, fast pulse

Treatment for Volume Shock

- Treat the cause.
- Rehydrate.
- Intravenous therapy may be needed, e.g., a blood transfusion.

Related Chapters

- Diagnosis and Treatments > Circulatory System > Dehydration and Volume Shock > Rehydration Plan

REHYDRATION PLAN

Oral Rehydration Solution

Only use oral rehydration if the patient is capable, or it may cause more harm than good, e.g., if the water goes into the airways.

Oral rehydration solutions are available commercially or can be easily made by combining 6 teaspoons sugar, 0.5 teaspoon salt, and 1 liter of drinkable water.

Ingest 50 to 200 ml/kg/24 hours (the stomach can only absorb 1 liter of liquid per hour).

If oral rehydration is not possible due to patient condition, intravenous therapy may be required.

BRAT

When the patient is able, advance to BRAT foods: bananas, rice, applesauce, toast, or crackers (plain).

Finally, give the patient solid foods.

DIABETES-RELATED ILLNESSES

Diabetes is a condition of high blood sugar levels in the body. Diabetics are more prone to infection, illness, and temperature-related injuries.

There are three main types of diabetes:

Type 1 occurs when the body does not produce enough insulin. The cause is unknown.

Type 2 occurs when cells do not respond to insulin properly. The cause is usually due to an unhealthy lifestyle, e.g., being overweight.

Gestational diabetes occurs in pregnant women who develop a high blood glucose level.

Diabetes Maintenance

- Back-up source of insulin
- Frequent munching
- Injectable glucagon
- Monitoring of maintenance of blood sugar levels
- Routine planning of meals

Prevention of Diabetes

- Maintain a healthy lifestyle

Related Chapters

Diagnosis and Treatment > Environmentally Induced

HYPOGLYCEMIA

Hypoglycemia is low blood sugar, and although not as common, it can also happen to non-diabetics. It can be caused by alcohol, birth defects, diabetes, excessive insulin, hormone deficiencies, infection, medications and poisons, organ failure, prolonged starvation, etc.

Symptoms of Hypoglycemia

Onset in minutes/hours:

- Anxiety
- Decreased mental status (AVPU)
- Cool and moist skin
- Elevated vital signs

Treatment for Hypoglycemia

- If unconscious, rub sugar (honey) under tongue and around gums.
- Complex carbohydrates if able to eat
- Glucose solution
- Hydration if able to drink

Related Chapters

- Must Read > Immediate First Aid > Critical First Aid > Mental Status: AVPU

HYPERGLYCEMIA

Hyperglycemia is excessive blood sugar, and although not as common, it can also happen to non-diabetics. It can be caused by critical illness, diabetes, drugs, etc.

Symptoms of Hyperglycemia

- Decreased mental status (AVPU)
- Flushed, dry skin
- Fruity smell on breath
- Intense thirst
- Loss of appetite
- Nausea
- Onset in days
- Progressive dehydration

Treatment for Hyperglycemia

- Adjusted insulin levels and diet
- Hydration

Related Chapters

- Diagnosis and Treatments > Circulatory System > Dehydration and Volume Shock > Dehydration

DIGESTIVE SYSTEM

ABDOMINAL PAIN

The acronym **ABDOMINAL** can help you to assess the cause of abdominal pains.

- **Associated symptoms:** What other symptoms are present, e.g., nausea, vomiting, fever, weakness, headache?
- **Blood:** Is there blood in the stool or vomit? How much? What color is it (red or darker)?
- **Description:** What does the pain feel like? Is it sharp or dull, constant or intermittent, localized or general, and is it getting worse?
- **Onset:** When did the pain start? Was it gradual or sudden? What makes it feel better (or worse)?
- **Menstruation:** Is it a female patient? Could her menstruation cycle have anything to do with it? Could she be pregnant?
- **Inspection:** Inspect the abdomen with palpation. Is there any tenderness?
- **Nutrition:** This includes food and hydration. What's gone in? What's come out?
- **Auscultation:** What sounds are his/her bowels making?
- **Losing volume:** Is the patient vomiting? Does the patient have diarrhea? If so, how much?

Treatment for Abdominal Pain

- Treat underlying problem if possible.
- Rehydrate if needed.
- Ginger
- Honey, water, and vinegar
- Peppermint tea

When to seek advanced medical care:

- Abdominal trauma
- Altered mental status
- Blood in vomit or stool other than small amount, e.g., hemorrhoid
- Diarrhea for over 24 hours
- Dehydration
- Fever
- Persistent pain
- Tenderness for over 24 hours
- Vomiting for over 24 hours

Related Chapters

- Must Read > Secondary Exam > Physical Exam
- Diagnosis and Treatments > Digestive System > Hemorrhoids
- Diagnosis and Treatments > Circulatory System > Dehydration and Volume Shock > Dehydration

ALCOHOL POISONING

Alcohol poisoning is the over-consumption of alcohol to dangerous levels.

It usually occurs when drinking large amounts of alcohol in a short time and can be life threatening.

Besides drinking of alcoholic beverages, it can also be caused by consuming household products that contain alcohol.

Symptoms of Alcohol Poisoning

- Confusion
- Hypothermia
- Reduced respiratory rate (less than eight breaths a minute)
- Seizures
- Skin discoloration (blue tinge or pale)
- Unconsciousness
- Vomiting

Treatment for Alcohol Poisoning

- Keep patient awake. A person who cannot be woken up is in danger of dying. Get to advanced medical help ASAP.
- All cases of alcohol poisoning should be referred to advanced medical help.
- Do not induce vomiting.
- Sit patient upright or lay them on their side if unable to sit.

Related Chapters

- Diagnosis and Treatment > Environmentally Induced > Cold and/or Water Induced > Hypothermia
- Diagnosis and Treatments > Head > Brain > Seizure

HANGOVERS

A hangover is the collection of unpleasant symptoms you experience after the consumption of alcohol. While drinking, it may be helpful to keep in mind that the more you drink the more likely and worse your hangover will be.

Symptoms of a Hangover

- Anxiety
- Dehydration
- Depression
- Dizziness
- Fatigue and weakness
- Headache
- Increased heart rate
- Irritability
- Light and sound sensitivity
- Muscle aches
- Nausea
- Shakiness
- Stomach pain
- Vomiting

Treatment for a Hangover

- Hangovers dissipate on their own within a day or two.
- Hydration (sports drinks are good)
- Honey (eat a few tablespoons)
- Sleep
- Analgesics (acetaminophen is preferred over NSAIDs)

Prevention of Hangovers

The obvious prevention is to not drink. Otherwise, try the following:

- Alternate alcoholic drinks with nonalcoholic beverages.
- Avoid darker-colored drinks.
- Before you go to sleep, drink electrolytic drinks and take a couple of Tylenol.
- Don't smoke or do other drugs while drinking.
- Eat before drinking.

APPENDICITIS

Appendicitis is inflammation of the appendix. Patients are usually under 40 years of age. No obvious cause has been proven.

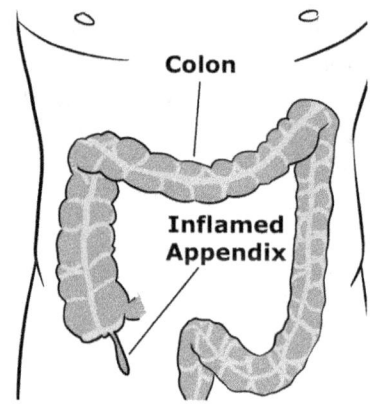

Symptoms of Appendicitis

- Discomfort in the area of the belly button which moves to lower right of the abdomen after 12 to 24 hours
- Abdominal swelling
- Constipation or diarrhea
- Difficulty passing gas
- Fever and chills
- Nausea
- Loss of appetite
- Pain worsening with coughs or walking
- Vomiting

Note: A sign of a ruptured appendix is pain that increases when you remove your hand after pressing it (rebound tenderness).

Treatment for Appendicitis

- Seek advanced medical care.
- Restrict patient to clear liquids in small amounts.
- Surgical removal of appendix if possible; ensure positive diagnosis as some conditions show similar symptoms to appendicitis, e.g., kidney diseases, ovarian cysts, pelvic inflammatory disease, tubal pregnancy, etc.
- If surgery is not possible, administer antibiotics.
- Antibiotic combination: Ciprofloxacin 500 mg every 12 hours and metronidazole 250 to 500 mg every 8 hours.

CONSTIPATION

Constipation is what occurs when a person suffers from infrequent or hard-to-pass bowel movements. Some common causes are lack of exercise, lack of opportunity to defecate, dehydration, lack of fiber, etc.

Symptoms of Constipation

- Cramping
- Hard, dry stool
- Inability/unwillingness to move bowels.

Treatment for Constipation

- Caffeine. This is a diuretic found in coffee, tea, etc. Drink an extra glass of water for every cup.
- Hydration. Two liters of water a day for adults.
- Increase fiber intake, e.g., bran, psyllium seed (Metamucil).
- Provide a comfortable environment to pass the stool, e.g., a private place and lots of time.
- Raw dehydrated flax seeds can help prevent traveler's constipation.
- Laxative
- Stool softener

DIVERTICULITIS

Diverticulitis is a common intestinal infection, usually occurring in people over 40. Pouches can form inside the lining of the colon known as diverticula. When these pouches fill with feces, it can lead to infection.

Symptoms of Diverticulitis

Symptoms may last hours, weeks, or even longer. The most common one is pain in the lower left of the belly, which may increase when moving. Pain could also be on the lower right, which is more common in those of Asian descent. Other symptoms include:

- Bloating and gas.
- Constipation or diarrhea (diarrhea less common).
- Fever and chills.
- Loss of appetite.
- Nausea.
- Vomiting.

Treatment for Diverticulitis

- Seek advanced medical care for further testing.
- Treat symptoms, e.g., compresses for belly pain, NSAIDs.
- Antibiotic combination: Ciprofloxacin 500 mg every 12 hours and metronidazole 7.5 mg/kg every 6 hours, maximum 4 g per day for 7 to 14 days.

Prevention of Diverticulitis

- High-fiber diet
- Regular bowel movements

FOOD POISONING

Food poisoning or food-borne illness results when infectious organisms (bacteria, viruses, and parasites) or their toxins are consumed.

Most cases of food poisoning are mild and resolve over time. Others, such as those caused by toxins from plants, may be more serious and advanced medical care may be needed.

Symptoms of Food Poisoning

- Confusion
- Dizziness
- Nausea
- Palpitations
- Vision disturbances
- Vomiting

Treatment for Food Poisoning

- Wash your mouth out as soon as possible.
- Make yourself vomit either with 2 fingers down your throat or Ipecac. When using Ipecac, only use the smallest amount that will cause you to vomit.
- Drink lots of clear fluids to help flush your system.
- Activated charcoal is preferable. If that is unavailable, mix tea and wood charcoal (not briquettes) and add milk of magnesia if available.
- Apple cider vinegar: Two tablespoons of apple cider vinegar in a glass of water, 4 times a day, sweeten if needed.
- Lemon juice: A glass of lemon juice 4 times a day, sweeten it if needed.

Related Chapters

- Diagnosis and Treatments > Environmentally Induced > Toxic Plants

GAS

Gas (flatus) is created in the stomach when the body breaks down food. Most people pass gas about 14 times a day. Excessive gas may be caused by certain foods or beverages, certain medications, swallowing too much air, or underlying medical problems, e.g., Crohn's disease.

Symptoms of Gas

- Bloated feeling
- Burping
- Flatulence
- Pain if gas is in the intestine

Treatment for Gas

- Treat underlying illness.
- Change diet.
- Simethicone, e.g., Gas-x, Mylicon
- Garlic
- Ginger

HEARTBURN

Heartburn (acid reflux, indigestion, pyrosis, GERD, etc.) is a burning sensation in the chest behind the breastbone. It is caused by stomach acid flowing back up into the gullet (the pipe that food moves down).

The pain may also radiate up to the throat.

Treatment for Heartburn

- Epigastric pain (upper central region of the abdomen) may be relieved by eating.
- Antacids, e.g., Mylanta, Rolaids, Tums
- Anti-ulcer meds, e.g., Famotidine, Omeprazole

Prevention of Heartburn

If you are prone to heartburn, consider the following:

- Don't eat within 2 hours of lying down.
- Eat smaller portions.
- Eat more slowly.
- Avoid heartburn triggers. These are different for different people, e.g., caffeine, chocolate, citrus, high-fat foods, onions, peppermint, tomatoes.

HEMORRHOIDS

Hemorrhoids are painful, swollen veins in the lower portion of the rectum that often protrude from the anus. They are more common during pregnancy and are caused by low fiber diets and/or too much pressure.

Symptoms of Hemorrhoids

- Bluish lump at the edge of the anal opening or inside the anal canal
- Inflammation, itching and redness to anus
- Pain while defecating and sitting
- Small amount of blood in stool

Treatment for Hemorrhoids

Hemorrhoids usually go away after a few weeks. If needed, you can try the following to soothe discomfort:

- Pads (cushioning)
- Hydrocortisone cream
- Specific soothing creams, e.g., Anusol
- Stool softeners to decrease further trauma

For severe cases the clot may need to be removed.

If advanced medical care is not available, a simple incision can be made to relieve pressure. This will not remove the hemorrhoid completely, and it may come back.

- Clean the area thoroughly with antiseptic.
- Use local anesthesia if available.
- Incise the skin over the hemorrhoid and drain the clotted

blood; only cut as deep as you have to in order to drain the blood.
- Relief should come very quickly.
- Be prepared to absorb any bleeding, e.g., gauze pads.
- Clean and dress.

HEPATITIS

Hepatitis is a condition occurring when the liver becomes inflamed. This impairs the body's ability to do many important things, including processing of toxins. Hepatitis can result in death.

There are many types of hepatitis, but hepatitis A, B, and C are the most common.

Advanced medical care is needed for precise diagnosis and treatment. If that is not available, field diagnosis and treatment are the same regardless of the type.

Symptoms of Hepatitis

- Dark urine
- Extreme fatigue
- Fever
- Grey stools
- Itchy feeling all over the body
- Jaundice (when the skin and the whites of the eyes turn yellow)
- Liver that is enlarged and/or tender to the touch
- Nausea
- Weight loss

Note: People with hepatitis may be symptomless.

Treatment for Hepatitis

Most cases of hepatitis will self-resolve after 2 to 6 weeks, but the patient should keep rested for 6 weeks after recovery.

- Avoid fatty foods and alcohol.
- Decrease protein intake.
- Eat. Force-feed if needed.

- Improve hydration, especially with herbal teas, vegetable broths, and diluted vegetable juices.
- Increase zinc intake.

Prevention of Hepatitis

- Hepatitis B vaccine
- Hygiene
- Not abusing drugs
- Safe sex

Related Chapters

- Must Read > Prevention > Vaccinations

NAUSEA AND VOMITING

Nausea is an uneasy feeling in the stomach which is often followed by vomiting. There are many possible causes including brain injury, drugs, emotional stress, motion sickness, morning sickness, overeating, pain (intense), smells, ulcers, underlying illnesses, etc. If vomiting does not cease within 24 hours, it may lead to volume shock.

Treatment for Nausea and Vomiting

- Fresh air
- Treating the underlying cause
- Anti-vomiting medication, e.g., ondansetron (Zofran)
- Dimenhydrinate (Dramamine) for motion sickness: 50 to 100 mg every 4 to 6 hours, to a maximum of 400 mg in 24 hours; the first dose should be taken 30 to 60 minutes before starting activity.
- Clove oil: Diffused clove oil is good for morning sickness. One drop on the roof of the mouth may help relieve nausea.
- Ginger: Most useful for motion sickness. Candied ginger is good to keep handy when traveling.

Related Chapters

- Diagnosis and Treatments > Circulatory System > Dehydration and Volume Shock > Volume Shock

PEPTIC ULCER

Peptic ulcers (stomach ulcers) are painful sores in the lining of the stomach. There are a variety of causes, including NSAIDs.

Symptoms of Peptic Ulcers

- Bloating
- Dark stool, i.e., blood (severe cases)
- Heartburn
- Nausea
- Pain (burning) in the middle or upper stomach between meals or at night, which can be severe
- Vomiting (blood in severe cases)

Treatment for Peptic Ulcers

Peptic ulcers are often self-healing. Medicinal treatment requires specific diagnosis and a combination of medicines.

- If experiencing severe and/or lingering symptoms, seek advanced medical care.
- Raw cabbage juice: 1 liter a day for 10 days.

Prevention of Peptic Ulcers

- Eat 4 or 5 small meals a day.
- Avoid alcohol, carbonated beverages, coffee, fruit juice, and milk.

WORMS

Worms are parasites which live inside the body. They are contagious, so immaculate hygiene is needed to prevent their spread.

Symptoms of Worms

- Diarrhea
- Gas or bloating
- Fatigue
- Itching in the anal area
- Nausea
- Passing a worm in your stool
- Stomach pains
- Weight loss
- Vomiting

Treatment for Worms

- Keep hands away from anus, e.g., when sleeping.
- Wash anus every morning.
- Vermicides, e.g., Vermox
- Garlic
- Honey, vinegar, and water. Drink lots of it regularly.
- Kerosene or gasoline. Drink a few tablespoons (kerosene is best). Only use if there is no other choice.
- Tannin tea (strong)

DIARRHEA

Diarrhea is a condition of frequent loose, watery stools.

Treatment for Diarrhea

Most cases of diarrhea will resolve itself within 24 hours if you restrict the patient to nothing but easily digested foods, i.e., applesauce, bananas, crackers, noodles, potatoes, rice, soups, and toast.

Traveler's diarrhea can last up to a week. Treatments include:

- Identifying and treating/preventing the cause.
- Monitoring and treatment to prevent dehydration.
- Rehydration plan.

It is best to just let diarrhea pass, but if you need to slow the symptoms, these medications can help:

- Anti-fever
- Antisecretory: Pepto Bismol every hour, max 120 ml/day.
- Loperamide: Imodium, 4 mg initial dose then 2 mg every 4 hours, max 16 mg/day.

Prevention of Diarrhea

- Avoid milk.
- Clean and/or peel fruits and vegetables.
- Cook food properly.
- Disinfect water.
- Practice good hygiene.

Alternative Remedies for General Diarrhea and Dysentery

- Brown rice water: Boil brown rice in double the amount of water with a pinch of salt. Strain and drink the water.
- Tea every two to three hours: Chamomile (strong), garlic and honey, peppermint, plantain seeds, tannin (strong for dysentery, will taste terrible), and ginger tea will decrease any abdominal cramps.

For severe cases when nothing else is available:

- Bones: Burn then grind them into a powder. Swallow the powder.
- Chalk: Consume school chalk.
- Activated charcoal is preferable. If that is unavailable, mix tea and wood charcoal (not briquettes) and add milk of magnesia if available.

Related Chapters

- Diagnosis and Treatments > Circulatory System > Dehydration and Volume Shock > Dehydration
- Diagnosis and Treatments > Circulatory System > Dehydration and Volume Shock > Rehydration Plan

MORE SERIOUS THAN DIARRHEA

Diarrhea in many cases is just diarrhea, but sometimes it is the sign of something more serious, e.g., appendicitis, cholera, colitis, intestinal bleeding, liver dysfunction.

Symptoms of Something More Serious than Diarrhea

- Black or grey-white stool
- Blood or mucus in the stool
- Diarrhea lasting more than 3 days
- Violent diarrhea violent for more than 24 hours
- Fever equal to or greater than 38 °C (101 °F)
- 'Rice water' diarrhea with fishy smell (indicates cholera)
- Severe vomiting
- Major abdominal distension and pain
- Moderate to severe dehydration

Treatment for Something More Serious than Diarrhea

- Seek advanced medical care.
- Treat cause if possible.
- Treat dehydration as described in related chapter.
- Do not give antimotility agents, e.g., loperamide (Imodium).

Antibiotics are not needed for recovery in most cases and should only be considered in severe cases. For traveler's diarrhea, research must be done on cases of antibiotic resistance depending on region.

- Antibiotic for cholera: Ciprofloxacin 1 g orally once, as an adjunct to fluid and electrolyte replacement.
- Antibiotic for cholera: Doxycycline 200 mg on the first day, given in 2 divided doses followed by 100 mg per day or 100 mg orally every 12 hours for severe cases.

- Antibiotic for infectious diarrhea: Ciprofloxacin 500 mg every 12 hours for 5 to 7 days.
- Antibiotic for traveler's diarrhea: Ciprofloxacin 500 mg every 12 hours for 3 to 7 days.
- Antibiotic for traveler's diarrhea: Sulfamethoxazole/trimethoprim

Related Chapter

- Diagnosis and Treatments > Circulatory System > Dehydration and Volume Shock > Dehydration

DYSENTERY

Dysentery is diarrhea which contains blood. It may be caused by an infection (viral, bacterial, or parasitic), ingestion of contaminated food or water, oral contact with contaminated objects or hands, poor hygiene, etc.

Symptoms of Dysentery

- Abdominal pain
- Diarrhea
- Feeling of incomplete defecation
- Fever

Treatment for Dysentery

- Drink lots of boiled water.
- Do not give antimotility agents, e.g., loperamide (Imodium).

Specific medications for dysentery depend on the type, i.e., amoebic or bacillary. The diagnosis of these is usually made in a lab with stool samples.

If there is no advanced medical care available and the dysentery does not self-resolve, a combination of an amoebicidal drug (to kill parasites) and an antibiotic (to treat bacterial infection) may help, e.g., ampicillin (antibiotic) 500 mg every 6 hours and metronidazole (systemic amoebicide) 750 mg 3 times a day for 5 to 10 days.

SALMONELLA

Salmonella is a type of food poisoning which can cause typhoid fever, paratyphoid fever, and salmonellosis.

The most common foods affected are beef, eggs, milk, and poultry, but anything has the potential to be infected and will often show no signs of contamination.

Apart from poorly handled food, salmonella can also be transmitted via drinks and animal feces (especially that of baby birds), rodents, reptiles, or any pet that has diarrhea.

Be sure to wash your hands after being in contact with any of these types of animals.

Symptoms of Salmonellosis

- Abdominal cramps
- Diarrhea
- Fever

Treatment for Salmonellosis

Salmonellosis usually subsides within a week.

- Treat symptoms.
- Monitor for dehydration.
- Antibiotic: Ciprofloxacin 500 mg every 12 hours for 10 days.

Prevention of Salmonella

Apart from general good hygiene, the following precautions can be taken:

- Avoid raw or unpasteurized dairy products.
- Cook foods well.
- Do not eat undercooked eggs, including those in homemade sauces/salad dressings (Caesar, hollandaise sauce, mayonnaise, etc.) or other foods (ice cream, tiramisu, etc.).
- Keep uncooked meats separate from produce, cooked foods, and ready-to-eat foods (cross-contamination).
- Wash or peel fruit and vegetables.

Related Chapters

- Diagnosis and Treatments > Circulatory System > Dehydration and Volume Shock > Dehydration

TYPHOID/PARATYPHOID FEVER

Typhoid fever is caused by either the salmonella typhi or paratyphi bacteria. For practical purposes, consider paratyphoid a less serious version of typhoid fever.

Regions of highest risk are Chile, India, Mexico, Pakistan, Peru, Southeast Asia, and Sub-saharan Africa.

It is possible for carriers to have no symptoms and carry/pass on the illness for years.

Vaccinations are available.

Symptoms of Typhoid and Paratyphoid Fever

- Abdominal pain
- Constipation
- Decreased appetite
- Decreased heart rate (bradycardia)
- Diarrhea (more common in young children)
- Fever as high as 40 °C (140 °F), slowly increasing over days and lasting 20 or so days before reducing again
- Generalized aches and pains
- Headaches
- Lethargy
- Reddish lesions on torso (rare)

Treatment for Typhoid and Paratyphoid Fever

Uncomplicated typhoid fever usually resolves within a month.

- Antibiotics can speed up recovery. Improvement will show within days, and recovery should follow within weeks. Exact diagnosis is made with a stool sample, and correct antibiotics are given accordingly.

- Relapses may occur after a week or two and are more common in those that take antibiotics. Relapses are treated in the same manner.
- Antibiotic: Ciprofloxacin 500 mg every 12 hours for 10 days.
- Antibiotics (other): Ampicillin, azithromycin.

Related Chapters

- Must Read > Prevention > Vaccinations

GENITOURINARY SYSTEM

KIDNEY INFECTION

If a urinary infection is left untreated, it may spread to the kidneys. If the kidney infection is not treated, it can lead to sepsis in the bloodstream.

Symptoms of a Kidney Infection

- Abdominal pain
- Bloody, cloudy, or foul urine
- Decreased mental status in the elderly
- One-sided back or flank pain
- Pain when urinating
- Persistent fever and chills

Treatment for a Kidney Infection

- Tests, e.g., a blood culture, should be done for a proper diagnosis so the correct antibiotic and dosage can be administered.
- Antibiotic: Cephalexin 500 mg every 6 hours for 14 days.

Related Chapters

- Must Read > Open Wounds, Skin Infections, and Sepsis > Open Wounds

KIDNEY STONES

Kidney stones are small and hard deposits made from mineral and acid salts which form inside the kidneys. They can be painful to pass, but usually no permanent damage is caused.

Kidney stones often form when urine becomes concentrated, so adequate hydration is a good preventative.

Symptoms of Kidney Stones

- Blood in urine
- Severe flank pain radiating to genitals

Treatment for Kidney Stones

- Hydration
- Wait for the stone to pass.
- Consider surgery if stone does not pass on its own.

PROSTATITIS

Prostatitis is an infection of the prostate gland. It is most common in men under the age of 50.

Symptoms of Prostatitis

Symptoms depend on the cause, e.g., bacterial, immune system disorder, prostate injury, etc. They may include:

- Difficulty urinating
- Flu-like symptoms (with bacterial prostatitis)
- Frequent urination (especially at night)
- Pain in the abdomen, groin, or lower back
- Pain when ejaculating
- Pain in the penis or testicles
- Pain in the perineum
- Pain when urinating
- Urgent need to urinate

Treatment for Prostatitis

- Seek advanced medical care for definitive diagnosis and treatment.
- Alpha blockers to ease symptoms
- NSAIDs
- Antibiotic for chronic bacterial prostatitis: Ciprofloxacin 500 mg every 12 hours for 28 days.
- Antibiotics, other: Cephalexin, levofloxacin, sulfamethoxazole/trimethoprim
- Avoid alcohol, caffeine, and acidic or spicy foods.
- Relieve pressure off the prostate, e.g., sit on a pillow.
- Soak in a warm bath.

URINARY TRACT INFECTIONS

A urinary tract infection (UTI) is when there is an infection of any of the organs that urine passes through before excretion of urine, i.e., kidneys, ureters, bladder, or urethra. If left untreated, it can lead to a kidney infection.

The most commonly known UTI is an infection of the bladder. It is most common in women, but men are susceptible also.

Causes of UTI include dehydration, lack of toilet use, poor hygiene, sexual transmission, etc.

Symptoms of Urinary Tract Infections

- Blood-tinged urine
- Frequent urge to urinate
- Painful, burning urination

Treatment for Urinary Tract Infections

- Cranberry juice
- Hydration
- Applying warmth to the bladder can be soothing.
- Phenazopyridine: This will eliminate painful urination. It may cause your urine to temporarily have a reddish-orange tinge.
- Antibiotic: Amoxicillin/clavulanate 500 mg every 12 hours for 3 to 7 days, or 875 mg every 12 hours for 3 to 7 days for serious cases.
- Antibiotic: Ciprofloxacin 250 mg every 12 hours for 3 days for uncomplicated cases (cystitis), or 250 mg every 12 hours for 7 to 14 days for moderate cases, or 500 mg every 12 hours for 7 to 14 days for severe cases.
- Antibiotic: Doxycycline 200 mg on the first day, given in 2

or 4 evenly divided doses, then 100 mg per day given once a day or in 2 divided doses for 3 to 7 days, or 100 mg every 12 hours for 3 to 7 days for severe cases.
- Antibiotics, other: Amoxicillin, ampicillin, levofloxacin, sulfamethoxazole/trimethoprim
- Alka-Seltzer and warm water poured over the urethra 3 times a day

Prevention of Urinary Tract Infections

- Cranberry juice
- Hydration
- Proper hygiene
- Safe sex
- Urinating immediately after sexual intercourse
- Urinating regularly
- Wearing cotton undergarments (increases air flow)
- Wiping from front to back after going to toilet

Related Chapters

- Diagnosis and Treatments > Genitourinary System > Kidney Infection

VAGINAL INFECTIONS

A vaginal yeast infection (monilia) is not a sexually transmitted disease and is, in fact, extremely common.

Symptoms of a Vaginal Yeast Infection

- Odorless, thick, white discharge reminiscent of cottage cheese
- Vaginal itchiness

Treatment for a Vaginal Yeast Infection

- Antifungal: Miconazole cream or suppository
- Antifungal for recurring cases: Fluconazole 150 mg once, repeated in 3 days if symptoms persist.

BACTERIAL VAGINOSIS

Bacterial vaginosis is a non-yeast vaginal infection caused by bacteria.

Trichomoniasis is also a non-yeast vaginal infection caused by protozoa.

Symptoms of Bacterial Vaginosis

- Foul odor

Treatment for Bacterial Vaginosis

- Vinegar and water douche (minor infections): 1 tablespoon of vinegar mixed with a liter of water, use until patient feels better, douche once daily.
- Antifungal: Metronidazole 500 mg every 8 hours for 5 to 7 days.
- Garlic: Insert a clove of garlic wrapped in gauze in the vagina for no longer than 8 hours. Ensure you leave some gauze to reach for easy removal.

Caution: Douching too often will actually cause yeast infections, so only use when needed.

PREGNANCY-RELATATED CONDITIONS

Pregnancy is the development of one or more fetuses in the womb. In a normal setting, it can be a blessing, and although complications can arise, the general procedure of birth has a high success rate.

In the case where there is no advanced medical care or facilities, it is best to avoid pregnancy.

During all stages of pregnancy, it is important that the patient has adequate nutrition.

Symptoms of Pregnancy

- Absent menstruation
- Backache
- Darkening of the nipples
- Fatigue
- Frequent urination
- Hemorrhoids
- Nausea and vomiting, i.e., morning sickness
- Stretch marks
- Tender breasts

- Varicose veins
- Visually pregnant

Symptoms of Impending Labor

An approximate due date can be calculated if the first day of the patient's last period is known. From that date, subtract 3 months and then add 7 days. For example: If the first day of her last period was November 7th and you subtract three months, you get August 7th. Then add seven days to get August 14th.

Expect the following near the due date:

- Change in abdominal appearance, i.e., the fetus repositions deep in the pelvis.
- Mucus-like and sometimes bloody discharge
- Contractions becoming more frequent
- Her water will break.

Note: Contractions may be irregular. This is known as false labor. Have the patient lie on her left side and hydrate well.

Related Chapters

- Diagnosis and Treatments > Digestive System > Nausea and Vomiting

DELIVERY

Construct a very sterile environment with gloves, clean sheets, etc. Avoid touching anything but the baby and the mother.

- Place a sheet under her buttocks and onto your lap, and a towel on her belly.
- Crowning is when the baby's head becomes visible.
- If the water has not broken, it will be visible and will rupture.
- Place two fingers along the edge of the vagina between the vagina and anus (perineum).
- Gently move your fingers from side to side to give the baby more room.
- The baby's head may move in and out with each contraction; this is okay.
- With each contraction the mother should take a deep breath and push while exhaling slowly.

Once the baby has been born, dry and wrap him/her in the towel on the mother's belly.

HYPEREMESIS GRAVIDARUM

Hyperemesis gravidarum is excessive vomiting during pregnancy.

Treatment for Hyperemesis Gravidarum

- Treat for dehydration.

Related Chapters

- Diagnosis and Treatments > Circulatory System > Dehydration and Volume Shock > Dehydration

MISCARRIAGE

When a woman miscarries, many times she will not pass all of the dead tissue relating to the pregnancy. On occasion, this tissue will become infected or cause excessive bleeding.

Symptoms of Miscarriage

- Bleeding or spotting from the vagina
- Pain simulating menstrual cramps

Treatment for Miscarriage

- Bed rest
- Watch for infection (fever and/or a foul discharge from the vagina).
- Antibiotics, other: Clindamycin, metronidazole

PREGNANCY-INDUCED HYPERTENSION

Pregnancy-induced hypertension usually occurs during the last month of pregnancy, most often with the mother's first baby. It can lead to seizures and can be life threatening.

Symptoms of Pregnancy-Induced Hypertension

- Elevated blood pressures
- Extreme swelling

Treatment for Pregnancy-Induced Hypertension

- Bed rest on the left side
- Consuming less salt
- Hydration (8 glasses of water a day)
- Consider blood pressure medication.

Related Chapters

- Diagnosis and Treatments > Head > Brain > Seizure

TUBAL PREGNANCY

Tubal (ectopic) pregnancy occurs when a fertilized egg wrongfully grows in the fallopian tube until it ruptures the tube. If left untreated, the fallopian tube will burst, causing internal bleeding which may lead to death.

Symptoms of Tubal Pregnancy

- Signs of normal pregnancy during the first few weeks
- Pelvic or belly pain which is possibly sharp on one side and then spreads through the abdomen, worsening with movement
- Vaginal bleeding

Treatment for Tubal Pregnancy

Advanced medical care is needed to treat an ectopic pregnancy. The earlier it is detected and treated, the less chance there is of permanent damage.

Related Chapters

- Diagnosis and Treatment > Circulatory System > Internal Bleeding

SEXUALLY TRANSMITTED INFECTIONS

There are many sexually transmitted infections, most of which are easily prevented with safe sex practices, i.e., monogamous relationships and/or the strict use of condoms.

Sexually transmitted infections are most commonly spread through sexual activity, but they may also be spread by fluid contact with an infected person, e.g., from a pregnant woman to an unborn child.

General Treatment for Sexually Transmitted Infections

If you suspect any sexually transmitted infection, seek advanced medical care for a definitive diagnosis.

Partners should also be tested, even if they have no symptoms.

After treatment, get retested to make sure the infection is gone.

Do not have sex until you are sure both you and your partner no longer have the disease.

General Prevention of Sexually Transmitted Infections

- Antibiotic prophylactic (preventative) if at high-risk, e.g., after sexual assault
- Condoms
- Monogamous relationships
- Regular STI checks
- Antibiotic for STI prophylaxis: Doxycycline 100 mg twice a day for 7 days.
- Antibiotic for STI prophylaxis, other: Metronidazole

CHLAMYDIA

Chlamydia is a common sexually transmitted bacterial infection. If left untreated, it can lead to pelvic inflammatory disease in women and epididymitis in men, which may cause sterility.

Chlamydia and gonorrhea often occur together.

Symptoms of Chlamydia

Symptoms do not always show, but if they do, you will probably notice them within a couple of weeks.

Symptoms of chlamydia in women:

- Abdominal pain with fever
- Bleeding between periods
- Burning and itching around vagina
- Pain during period, sex, and/or urination
- Vaginal discharge that may have an odor

Symptoms of chlamydia in men:

- Burning and itching around penis opening
- Discharge from tip of penis (clear or cloudy)
- Pain and swelling around the testicles
- Pain when urinating

Treatment for Chlamydia

The patient's sexual partner(s) should also be evaluated and treated if needed.

- Antibiotics should solve the problem within a couple of weeks.

- **Antibiotic:** Azithromycin single-dose is a preferred regimen.
- **Antibiotic for uncomplicated urethral, endocervical, or rectal infection:** Doxycycline 100 mg twice a day for 7 days.
- **Antibiotics, other**: Amoxicillin, azithromycin, levofloxacin, tetracycline

Related Chapters

- Diagnosis and Treatments > Genitourinary System > Sexually Transmitted Infections > Gonorrhea

GENITAL HERPES

Genital herpes is a common, highly contagious, and often reoccurring sexually transmitted infection usually caused by the herpes simplex virus, which is the same virus that causes cold sores.

Symptoms of Genital Herpes

Not every person will show symptoms, but those that do will usually experience symptoms within two weeks of infection. They will appear wherever the infection entered your body, e.g., buttocks, mouth, penis, vagina, etc.

Common symptoms of genital herpes:

- Pain or itching (first sign)
- Small, red bumps or tiny white blisters (showing a few days after the pain/itching)
- Ulcers then scabs forming as the ulcers heal

Other symptoms of genital herpes:

- Fever
- Headache
- Muscle aches
- Pain in genital area
- Pain when urinating

Treatment for Genital Herpes

There is no cure for genital herpes, but anti-viral medication can help prevent reoccurring cases and ease symptoms.

- Antivirals: Acyclovir or famciclovir 200 mg every 4 hours for 10 days.

Related Chapters

- Diagnosis and Treatments > Head > Mouth and Teeth > Cold Sores

GONORRHEA

Gonorrhea (the clap, the drip, gonococcal) is an easily spread sexually transmitted infection.

If gonorrhea is left untreated, it can lead to (amongst other things) pelvic inflammatory disease in women and epididymitis in men which may make them sterile.

Gonorrhea and chlamydia often occur together.

Symptoms of Gonorrhea

Not everyone who contracts gonorrhea will show symptoms, but those that do will usually experience symptoms within two weeks of infection. Gonorrhea may be confused with a yeast infection. Seek professional medical advice to be sure.

Symptoms of gonorrhea in women:

- Abdominal (lower) or pelvic pain
- Bleeding between periods
- Burning when urinating
- Conjunctivitis
- Discharge from vagina (greenish-yellow or whitish)
- Spotting after intercourse
- Vulvitis (swelling of the vulva)

If oral sex was performed:

- Burning in the throat
- Swollen throat glands

Symptoms of gonorrhea in men:

- Men are more likely to show symptoms than women.
- Burning when urinating

- Discharge from penis (greenish yellow or whitish)
- Painful or swollen testicles

If oral sex was performed:

- Burning in the throat
- Swollen throat glands

Treatment for Gonorrhea

- Seek advanced medical care for a definitive diagnosis, e.g., swab or urine test.
- Partners should also be tested, even if they have no symptoms.
- After treatment, get retested to make sure it is gone.
- Do not have sex until you are sure both you and your partner no longer have the disease.
- Antibiotic for uncomplicated urethral and cervical gonococcal infections: Ciprofloxacin 250 mg one time.
- Consider treating concurrent chlamydia infection, e.g., single-dose azithromycin.

Related Chapters

- Diagnosis and Treatments > Genitourinary System > Sexually Transmitted Infections > Chlamydia
- Diagnosis and Treatments > Genitourinary System > Vaginal Infections
- Diagnosis and Treatments > Head > Eyes > Conjunctivitis

PELVIC INFLAMMATORY DISEASE

Pelvic inflammatory disease is most often caused by a sexually transmitted infection such as chlamydia or gonorrhea. It is an infection of a woman's pelvic organs, i.e., cervix, fallopian tubes, ovaries, and womb. If left untreated it may lead to infertility, ectopic pregnancy, chronic pelvic pain, etc.

Symptoms of Pelvic Inflammatory Disease

- Pain and fever which may come with a quick onset
- Irregular periods
- Fever
- Foul vaginal discharge
- Pain on both sides of the lower abdomen
- Painful sex
- Painful urination

Treatment for Pelvic Inflammatory Disease

- Antibiotic: Doxycycline 100 mg every 12 hours for 14 days.
- Antibiotics, other: Azithromycin, levofloxacin, metronidazole, tetracycline

INTEGUMENTARY SYSTEM

ABSCESSES

A skin abscess (boil) is a bacterial skin infection that starts in a hair follicle or oil gland and forms a pocket of puss. It may be caused by a cyst, infected wound, etc.

They most commonly appear on the armpits, buttocks, face, neck, and shoulders. When there are a group of boils, it is known as a carbuncle.

Symptoms of an Abscess

Hard, red, painful lump which becomes softer, larger, and more painful. Pus forms on the top.

Signs of a severe infection:

- Fever
- Multiple abscesses
- Surrounding skin becomes infected (inflamed, red, etc.)
- Swollen lymph nodes

Treatment for an Abscess

For treatment of an abscess on the eye or mouth:

- Do not forcefully pop the abscess, e.g., with a needle.
- Warm water soaks and compresses
- Within 10 days of soaks, the boil should burst.
- Clean very well with antiseptic.
- Apply a topical antibiotic and cover.
- Continue cleaning and compresses until wound heals.

If spontaneous drainage does not happen within 10 days, an incision must be made.

- Ice the area to numb the skin.
- Pierce the skin where the abscess is closest to the skin's surface to drain the pus.
- Immediate relief will be felt.
- Apply a topical antibiotic and cover.

Related Chapters

- Diagnosis and Treatments > Head > Eyes > Stye
- Diagnosis and Treatments > Head > Mouth and Teeth > Dental Abscess

ACNE

Acne (pimples, blackhead, whiteheads, zits) occur when the sebaceous glands produce sebum (oily matter) and block the pores in the skin. This cultivates bacteria which break out as acne, usually on the back, face, and/or neck. The exact root cause is unknown, but diet (including food allergies), hormonal imbalance, and stress are thought to play a role.

Treatment for Acne

Most of the time, acne will go away on its own.

Alternative remedies are highly recommended before other medications.

- There are many creams available.
- Antibiotics can be used for serious cases.
- Antibiotic: Doxycycline 200 mg on the first day given in 2 divided doses, then 100 mg per day or 100 mg every 12 hours for severe cases.
- Antibiotics, other: Tetracycline
- Acidophilus (found in yogurt or as a capsule)
- Calendula (found in marigold petals)
- Garlic: Cut a clove of garlic in half and rub it over the affected area. Do it regularly.
- Honey (raw): Dab it onto affected areas; wait 15 minutes and then rinse it off.

Prevention of Acne

- Eat healthy and keep well hydrated.
- Keep pores clean.
- Minimize stress.

BLISTERS AND HOT SPOTS

A blister is typically a protective pocket of clear fluid (plasma) underneath the layers of the skin. If they are filled with blood, they are called blood blisters, and if they become infected, they will fill with puss.

They can be caused by cold, exposure to chemicals, friction, heat, etc.

The most common and troublesome blisters are those found on the feet which are caused by friction and heat while hiking or engaging in similar activities.

Before a blister forms, the area will often get red and painful. This is known as a hot spot. Treat it before it becomes a blister.

Treatment for Hot Spots

- A hot spot can simply be covered, e.g., Band-Aid.
- Ideally, raise the area around it slightly and then cover it.

Treatment for Blisters

- In controlled environments, the blister should be left intact. The skin will keep it protected from infection.
- Pad it like a hotspot.

Draining a blister:

If there is a chance of the blister rupturing, it is often better to drain it manually so you can clean and dress it.

- Clean the area around blister.
- Sterilize a needle and pierce the side of the blister.
- Let the fluid drain.

- Apply antibiotic ointment.
- Cover and monitor.

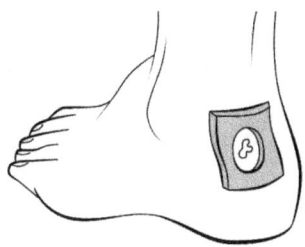

Prevention of Friction Blisters

- Proper footwear
- Sock liners
- Cover blister-prone areas with a Fixamol, a Band-aid, etc.
- Change wet/sweaty socks.
- Foot powders to keep feet dry

BRUISES

A bruise usually occurs from some kind of trauma which ruptures the blood vessels. They are somewhat painful to the touch and may change color from blackish-blue to brown to yellow.

Treatment for Bruises

- RICES
- In later stages, stretching may help.

Related Chapters

- Diagnosis and Treatments > Musculoskeletal System > Musculoskeletal Injuries in General

CHICKENPOX

Chickenpox (varicella) is a contagious virus causing a red, itchy rash. It is usually not harmful, (more harmful to people over 12 years), and once you have gotten it once you are not likely to get it again.

In some cases, the virus can reactivate, causing shingles.

Chickenpox is most contagious from a couple of days before the rash appears until all the blisters have crusted over. This crusting over usually takes about 10 days from the initial symptoms.

Vaccines are available.

Symptoms of Chickenpox

- Fever
- Headache
- Lethargy
- Loss of appetite
- Sore throat
- Itchy that rash appears a day or two after initial appearance of the above symptoms

Treatment for Chickenpox

- Treat rash with compresses, oatmeal baths, etc.
- Treat fever.
- Diphenhydramine
- For serious cases, consider the chickenpox vaccine, especially if over 12 years old, pregnant, or immunocompromised.

Related Chapters

- Diagnosis and Treatment > Integumentary System > Shingles

ECZEMA

Eczema is an irritation of the skin resulting in an itchy rash. It is not contagious.

It usually occurs when someone comes into contact with a known trigger; avoiding these triggers is the best defense.

The triggers are different depending on the person, but some common ones are allergies, animals, coarse materials, foods, soaps, respiratory infections, temperature, etc.

Stress can make the symptoms worse.

Symptoms of Eczema

- Change in skin pigmentation
- Dry, thickened, or scaly skin
- Itchy rash
- A crusty oozing can appear in infants.

Treatment for Eczema

- Avoid irritants.
- Avoid scratching.
- Apply cold compresses to help with itching.
- Moisturize, particularly while the skin is damp, e.g., after bathing.
- Diphenhydramine (helps with itching)
- Corticosteroids (for serious cases)
- Cyclosporine (last resort)
- Baths or compresses: Oatmeal, Epson salts, sea salts, or sulfur bath salts.

SHINGLES

Shingles (herpes zoster) is a reactivation of the chickenpox virus (varicella).

Vaccines are available.

Symptoms of Shingles

The telltale sign of shingles is a stripe of itchy/painful blisters wrapping around one side of the torso; this rash may appear elsewhere.

- Fatigue
- Fever
- Headache
- Sensitivity to light

Treatment for Shingles

Shingles will self-resolve within 2 to 6 weeks, but it can reoccur.

- Cool compresses
- Seek advanced medical care if pain and rash is near an eye or widespread.
- **Antivirals:** Acyclovir, famciclovir, valacyclovir.

Related Chapters

- Diagnoses and Treatments > Integumentary System > Chickenpox

SPLINTERS

A splinter is a piece of a larger object lodged inside the body, e.g., wood, glass, animal spine, metal.

A splinter is minor to begin with, usually just causing discomfort or minor pain, but if left untreated it may lead to infection or perhaps even internal damage.

Symptoms of a Splinter

- Abscess
- Bumps under the skin
- Cyst
- Discoloration beneath the skin
- Pain
- Puncture wound
- Wound that won't heal

Treatment for Splinters

- Clean the area.
- Using tweezers (or similar), pull the splinter out along the same angle that it entered the skin; a magnifying glass may help.
- If needed, place a thin slice of garlic over the splinter and hold on with a bandage. It should help the splinter work its way out after a few hours.
- If that doesn't work, carefully cut the skin that lies over it, just enough to expose the splinter.
- Clean the area.

Related Chapters

- Diagnosis and Treatments > Integumentary System > Abscesses

FISHHOOKS

If you cannot easily slide a fishhook out, it may be because of the barb.

Treatment for Fishhooks

Press down on the skin where the barb is and then pull it out.

Clean and dress.

If pulling back does not work:

- Put it further in until the barb comes out.
- Cut off the barbed end, e.g., using a wire cutter and remove the hook.

TINEA/RINGWORM

Tinea (ringworm) is a common fungal infection on the skin. Athlete's foot, jock itch, ringworm, scalp ringworm, etc., are all just forms of tinea in different places. It is usually not serious, but it can be irritating, and if not treated it may last for years. It is contagious.

One symptom is a skin rash that forms a ring—hence the name ringworm. It has nothing to do with worms, which are intestinal parasites.

Symptoms of Tinea

- Bald patches if on a hairy area
- Raised, itchy patch that is darker on the outside
- Blistering and oozing caused by scratching

Treatment for Tinea

For treatment of tinea on the feet, see athlete's foot.

- Avoid tight-fitting clothing on irritated areas.
- Keep skin as dry as possible.
- Wash regularly.
- Wash sheets daily.
- Drying powders, e.g., talcum powder
- Antifungals: Miconazole, clotrimazole
- Garlic: Cut in half and rub on area a few times a day.

Related Chapters

- Diagnosis and Treatments > Digestive System > Worms

ATHLETE'S FOOT

Athlete's foot (tinea pedis) is tinea/ringworm on the feet. It usually occurs between the toes but can also appear anywhere on the feet and hands. Keeping feet clean and dry, wearing footwear in public showers, etc., are the best ways to prevent contraction.

Athlete's foot can be caused by cuts on feet and hands, having wet feet for prolonged periods (including perspiration), sharing shoes or socks, spending long hours in closed shoes, wet surfaces, etc.

Symptoms of Athlete's Foot

- Discolored nails
- Flaking of skin
- Fluid drainage from surfaces traumatized by repeated scratching
- Itching and burning
- Reddened skin
- Oozing caused by scratching

Treatment for Athlete's Foot

- Keep feet clean and dry.
- Drying powders, e.g., talcum powder
- Avoid anti-itching creams as they keep the area moist and may delay healing.
- Antifungals: Miconazole, clotrimazole
- Garlic: Crush a couple of cloves into warm water for a 30-minute foot bath.

NAIL INJURIES

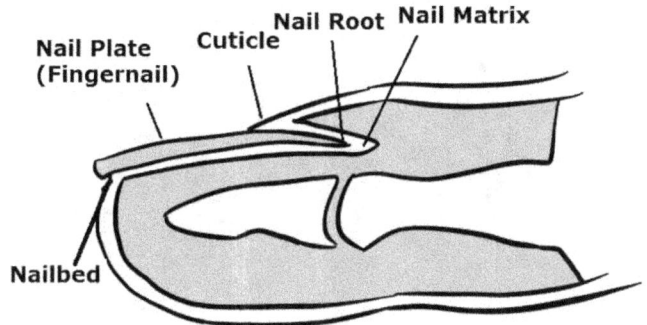

Nail plate: The hard covering of the end of your digit (the part what most people consider to be the nail)

Nail bed: The skin under the nail plate

Nail matrix: Part of the nail under the cuticle (the half-moon)

NAIL AVULSION

This is when the nail plate is ripped off by some sort of trauma.

Treatment for Nail Avulsion

A completely torn-off nail will take 4 to 5 months to grow back.

- Numb the area.
- Clean and dress with non-adherent dressing. Use antiseptic liberally.
- Change dressing frequently.
- If the nail is still attached to the nail bed by a small amount, remove it.
- Consider using the nail as a protective covering on the nail bed.
- Do not scrape off loose edges.

INGROWN TOENAIL

An ingrown toenail is when the nail grows in a way that it cuts into the skin at the end or side of the toe. It requires downward pressure by a shoe, so it does not occur in people that habitually do not wear shoes. If left untreated, it can lead to infection and/or other complications.

Symptoms of an Ingrown Toenail

- Redness
- Pain
- Swelling
- Warmth in the toe

Treatment for an Ingrown Toenail

- Do not repeatedly cut the nail.
- Foot soaks in warm water, 4 times a day.
- During the soak, gently massage the side of the nail fold to help reduce the inflammation.
- Wash with soap and water twice a day.
- Keep clean and dry during the rest of the day.
- Wear sandals if possible but definitely not heels.

After each soak:

- Roll up a small bit of clean gauze so it is like the wick of a candle.
- Lift up the troublesome corner of the nail.
- Stick the gauze between the nail and the skin. The idea is to keep it elevated until it grows out. Pain is normal.
- Try putting it further in after each soak.
- Change it every day.

Prevention of Ingrown Toenails

- Don't cut nails too short.
- Don't wear shoes that are too tight or too loose.

CRUSH INJURIES

Crush injuries are caused by trauma such as striking with a hammer, slamming in a door, etc.

Symptoms of a Crush Injury to the Nail

- Bruising (brown or blue)
- Blood (deep blue to black)
- Pain

Treatment for a Crush Injury to the Nail

A bruise will heal in time.

For significant blood under the nail, consider making a hole to relieve pressure:

- Using a hot paper clip or similar, make a hole in the nail plate.
- Dry, splint, and bandage for at least 48 hours.

MUSCULOSKELETAL SYSTEM

MUSCULOSKELETAL INJURIES IN GENERAL

There are two types of musculoskeletal injuries: stable and unstable. Whether an injury is stable or unstable will determine the basic treatment. Injury symptoms will define whether it is unstable or stable.

Symptoms of Stable and Unstable Musculoskeletal Injuries

The following symptoms may occur in both stable and unstable musculoskeletal injuries:

- Bruising/discoloration
- Pain
- Pop/snap
- Swelling
- Tenderness

Symptoms of Unstable Musculoskeletal Injuries

The following symptoms will occur only in unstable musculoskeletal injuries:

- Angulations/deformity
- Crepitus
- Feeling of instability
- Impaired CSM
- Reduced ability to bear weight

Treatment for Stable Injuries

- RICES

Treatment for Unstable Injuries

If there is severe deformity or loss of CSM, then the body part must be repositioned back towards its correct anatomical position unless a significant increase in pain or physical resistance is met.

In all other cases, the body part can be splinted in position.

RICES

RICES is an acronym for a common treatment of musculoskeletal injuries.

- **Rest:** Do your best to cease using the limb.
- **Ice:** Apply a cold compress (or similar) 4 times a day for approximately 20 minutes during the first 48 hours of the injury occurring.
- **Compression:** Apply a compression bandage after each cold therapy. Lightly pad the area, then wrap it starting below the joint and working your way up beyond it. The wrap should be as tight as possible without causing discomfort or impaired CSM.
- **Elevation:** Elevate the affected limb above the heart.
- **Stabilization:** Depending on the seriousness of the injury, a splint or cast may be needed.

If the injury is unstable, then a splint/cast is definitely necessary. The joint should be immobilized.

Impaired CSM

CSM stands for circulation, sensation, and movement. Testing for impaired CSM can help in diagnosing problems as well as ensuring that correct treatment is being given.

Circulation. Color, temperature and capillary refill:

- **Color:** Is the skin discolored?
- **Temperature:** Is the skin warm or cold?
- **Capillary refill:** Check perfusion.

Sensation. Have the patient close his/her eyes, then move a part of his/her body. Can the patient tell you which part you are moving?

Lightly tap with both dull (e.g., finger) and sharp (e.g., safety pin) sensations. Can the patient tell the difference?

Motion. Can the patient move the part of the body you are testing?

Related Chapters

- Diagnosis and Treatments > Musculoskeletal System > Dislocations
- Diagnosis and Treatments > Musculoskeletal System > Immobilization
- Must Read > Immediate First Aid > Critical First Aid > Circulation

IMMOBILIZATION

Immobilizing a body part means to prevent it from moving or bearing weight. This will stabilize the body part and allow it to rest.

Any injury that requires immobilization should be referred to advanced medical care when possible.

Immobilize the joints above and below the fracture, e.g., if it is the forearm, the elbow and the wrist are included in the splint.

For joint injuries, immobilize the bone above and below.

Immobilize joints in a position for normal function:

- **Ankles:** 90-degree angle to the leg
- **Elbows:** 90-degree angle to the upper arm
- **Fingers:** Slightly flexed, as if holding an apple
- **Legs:** Basically straight with a slight bend in the knee
- **Wrists:** Straight or extended slightly upward

Collars

Collars stabilize and support the neck and prevent further injury by limiting head movement. A collar can be improvised from a fanny pack, rolled towels, foam mat, etc.

Mobility Aids

These are things such as crutches, walking sticks, wheelchairs, etc. Aids like crutches and walking sticks can be easily improvised using any pole-type item.

Slings

Slings are used to immobilize an arm injury, including a wrist or shoulder. They are often used together with a cast or splint on the arm.

Triangular Bandage Sling and Swath

A triangular bandage can be improvised from many different materials, but having one or two of them in your first aid kit will save you some trouble. Also, a triangular bandage can be used in a variety of ways, e.g., to stop bleeding, tying something.

- Drape the triangular bandage under one arm and over the opposite shoulder.
- Tie the two ends of the cloth behind the neck.
- Pin the remaining elbow corner up onto the body of the sling.
- Use another bandage or similar to secure the arm to the chest.

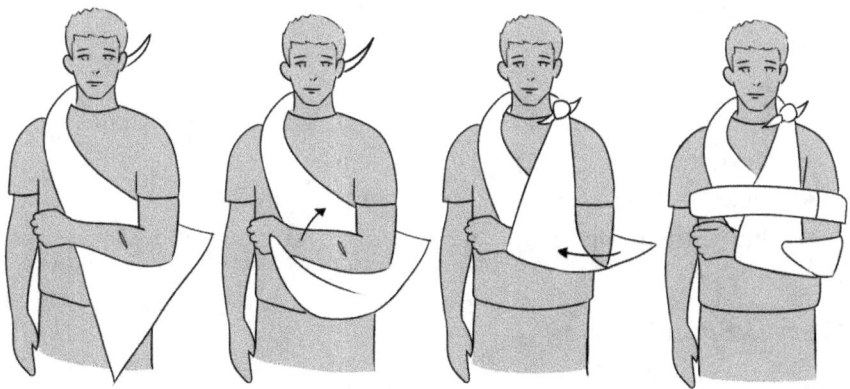

Shirt Slings

If wearing a long shirt, pin it to the chest.

If wearing a short-sleeved shirt, fold the bottom up over the injured arm and secure in place.

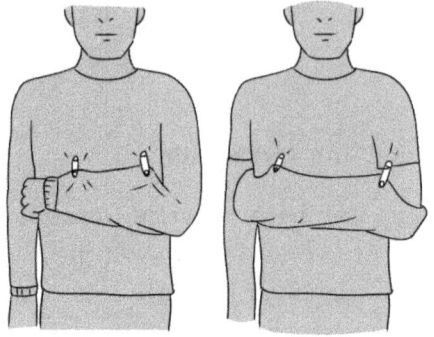

Splints

Splints are commonly improvised until a cast can be fitted. In the case of small fractures, splints may be the only thing used. Even in more serious injuries a splint can be used if a cast is not possible, and as long as proper care is taken, the injury will heal just as well.

Commercial field splints are readily available (SAM Splints), but they can also be improvised with a great number of readily available materials, e.g.:

- Body parts, e.g., adjacent digit (finger or toe), arm to chest, the patient's other leg.
- Sticks or straight, stiff materials from equipment.
- Pliable materials, e.g., strips of cloth, parachute cord.

General Splinting Tips

When constructing a splint, remember the following:

- Make it adjustable (and adjust when needed).
- It should be lightweight.
- Monitor CSM before and after splinting.
- Pad well.

- Sandwich the limb.

Example splint pictures from left to right: Ankle, leg, wrist.

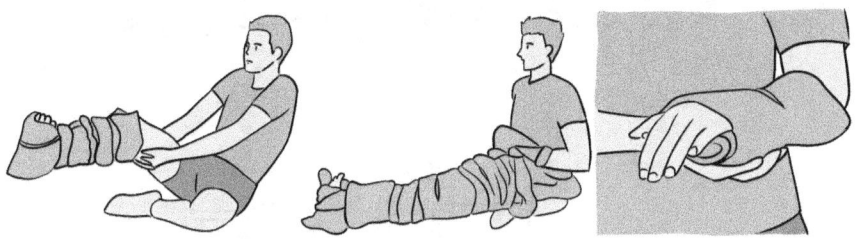

Taping

Taping is good for immobilizing while healing as well as preventing injuries, e.g., during sporting activities.

If taping around a whole body part (circumferential wrapping), e.g., for anchors, ensure swelling does not impair CSM. It is best to tape after swelling has gone down.

General Taping Tips

- Anchor points are those to which tape can stick.
- Avoid leaving gaps as they can lead to blisters.
- Duct tape can be used in emergencies, but it does not breathe well.
- Ensure your skin is dry.
- Follow the contour of the skin.
- Keep your limb in a neutral position.
- Overlap a half-width on each strip.

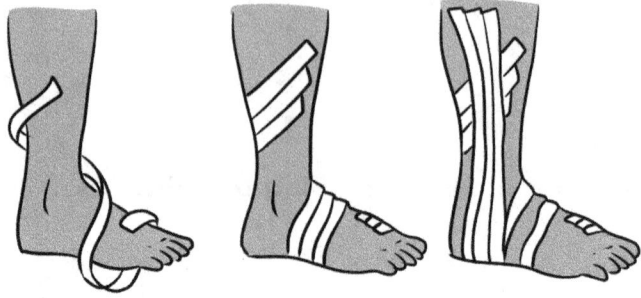

Taping an ankle.

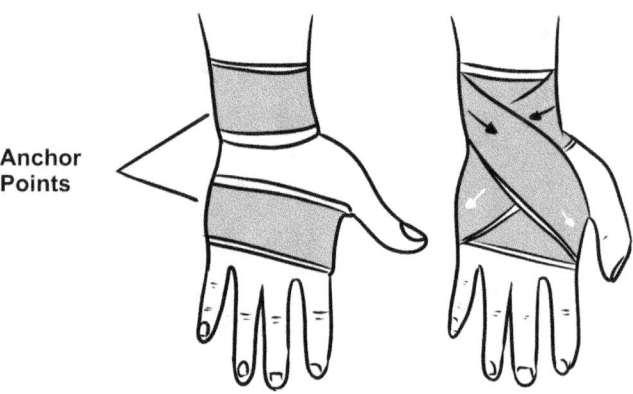

Taping a wrist.

Related Chapters

- Must Read > Secondary Exam > Physical Exam > Spinal Stabilization
- Diagnosis and Treatments > Musculoskeletal System > Musculoskeletal Injuries in General

AMPUTATIONS

Amputation is a last-resort procedure to remove all or part of an extremity in an effort to save a life in the case of severe injuries.

When to Amputate

- Cancerous tumors
- Extensive injury from trauma or burns
- Gangrene
- Serious infection that does not get better with antibiotics
- Severe frostbite

Where to Amputate

- At areas of reddened (infection) or blackened (gangrene) skin
- Where the bone has been crushed beyond repair
- Where the extremity is no longer sensitive to touch
- Where the extremity loses normal temperature
- Where the extremity loses pulse

Note: The closer to the body that the amputation is performed, the more dangerous it is.

Amputation Procedure

- Sedate the patient.
- Use antiseptics on the damaged area.
- Consider a tourniquet to prevent massive blood loss. Amputate the limb and preserve enough living tissue to cover the exposed end of the bone.
- Remove debris and bits of shattered bone.
- Tie off any bleeding blood vessels.

- Shorten and smooth the bone.
- Stitch remaining muscle to the bone lining if possible.
- Before closing completely, place a drain.
- Adequately close the wound with sutures or staples.
- Change dressings regularly.

Related Chapters

- Must Read > Immediate First Aid > Critical First Aid > Severe Bleeding

BACKACHE

Back pain is a common occurrence and usually feels like an ache, tension, or stiffness in your back. It can be caused from a variety of things, e.g., bad posture, incorrect lifting, pinched nerve, unusual movement (bending or twisting), etc. Sometimes it occurs for no apparent reason, e.g., you just wake up with a bad back. People with excess weight (including those who are pregnant) are more at risk.

Back pain is not generally caused by a serious condition, and in most cases, it gets better within 12 weeks. It can usually be successfully treated by taking painkillers, improving posture, and keeping mobile.

Treatment for a Backache

Back pain will usually go away within 12 weeks.

- Hot or cold compresses
- Unless incapacitated, continue with daily activities; excessive inactivity will make it worse.
- Muscle relaxers
- Practice correct posture.

PNEUMOTHORAX

Pneumothorax occurs when a lung is punctured and becomes decompressed, usually from a rib fracture.

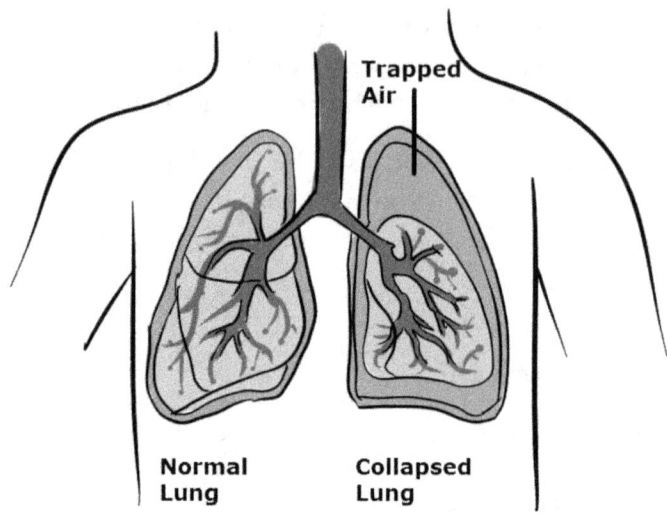

Symptoms of Pneumothorax

- Crackly or no sound from lungs
- Cyanosis (bluish skin)
- Pain with breathing
- Signs of shock
- Swollen neck veins

Treatment for Pneumothorax

Only treat if it becomes life threatening. This is definitely only for a last-resort do-or-die situation. Even if this operation is successful, the patient may not recover from the wound.

The aim of this is to create a way for the air to escape but not go back in, i.e., a one-way valve.

You need to make an incision in the collapsed lung, between the nipple and the top of the shoulder, just above the third rib.

- Clean the site.
- Make the incision no wider than a pencil, just deep enough to hear the air pass through.
- Tape three sides of a plastic bag or similar (cling film) over the incision.
- Fluid will build up in the lung. Drain it with a tube.

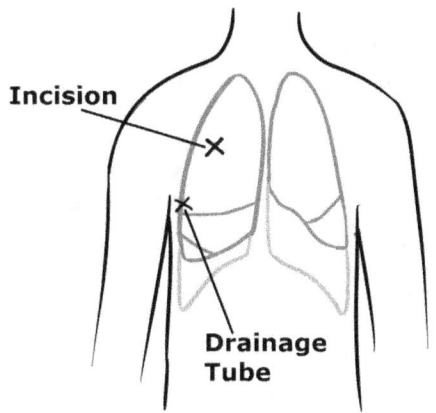

Related Chapters

- Diagnosis and Treatments > Musculoskeletal System > Fractures > Fractured Ribs
- Diagnosis and Treatments > Circulatory System > Dehydration and Volume Shock

TETANUS

Tetanus is an infection that targets the nerves serving muscle tissue.

It can be caused by any break in the skin, but puncture wounds are particularly vulnerable, e.g., animal bite, rusty nail, splinter.

Tetanus can be deadly, but there are vaccinations available.

Symptoms of Tetanus

Initial (may not present for up to 2 weeks):

- Difficulty swallowing
- Involuntary muscle contractions
- Irritability
- Lockjaw
- Sore muscles (especially near the site of injury)
- Weakness

Progressive:

- Fever
- High blood pressure
- Involuntary back arching
- Irregular heartbeat
- Muscle spasms
- Respiratory distress

Treatment for Tetanus

- Dim lights.
- Reduce noise.
- Rehydration
- Muscle relaxants: Valium in severe cases
- Antibiotics: Metronidazole, penicillin

DISLOCATIONS

A dislocation occurs when a bone is pulled out of the joint and is often a reoccurring injury. It can be caused either by a direct injury or an indirect injury.

Direct injuries: Caused by forces generated from outside the body, e.g., getting hit or crashing into a blunt object.

Indirect injuries: Caused by a force from within the body, e.g., injury from an abnormal twisting motion.

Symptoms of a Dislocation

- Bruising
- Pain and/or numbness
- Swelling
- Visibly abnormal
- Unusable

Treatment for a Dislocation

The dislocation may correct itself. This is called subluxation and is treated with RICES.

Dislocations that do not correct themselves require reduction and then stabilization.

Related Chapters

- Diagnosis and Treatments > Musculoskeletal System > Musculoskeletal Injuries in General
- Diagnosis and Treatments > Musculoskeletal System > Immobilization

REDUCTIONS

Reductions are safe to use on dislocations caused by an indirect force if the dislocation is of the shoulder, patella, or digits.

Everything else should be splinted in position unless there is no advanced medical care available in the foreseeable future.

Perform a reduction as soon as possible. Discontinue if pain significantly increases or physical resistance is encountered.

Use RICES after any successful reduction.

Any reduction that doesn't work after three attempts should be referred to advanced medical care.

Anti-inflammatories or muscle relaxers such as cyclobenzaprine (Flexeril) may be helpful.

Traction

Traction is a procedure in which you pull the dislocated bone away from the joint in order to give the bone room to slip back into place.

Hold the affected joint in a steady fashion.

Slowly pull the bone away from the joint.

Shoulder Reduction

There are two ways in which a dislocated shoulder can be reduced.

Whichever one you choose, and whether or not the reduction is successful, sling and swathe the arm so the elbow is alongside the body.

Pain and swelling are extremely likely.

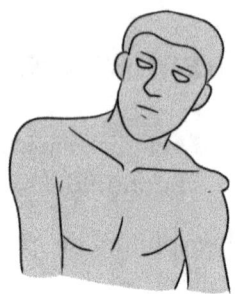

Shoulder reduction method one:

- Lay the patient on his/her back and sit next to the dislocated shoulder.
- Apply traction to the shoulder.
- While keeping the elbow at a 90-degree angle, gradually rotate the arm until it is in a baseball-throwing position.
- If successful, it will "pop" back into place.

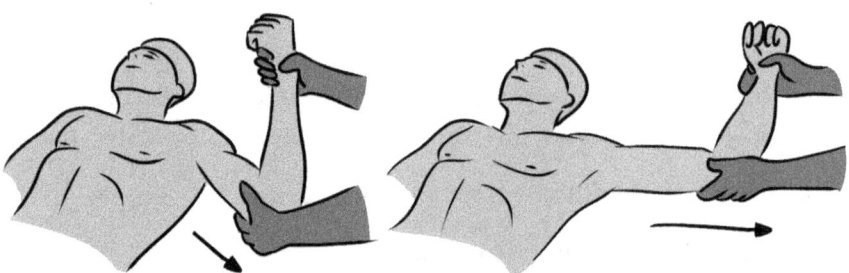

Shoulder reduction method two:

- Lay the patient facedown with the affected arm hanging unsupported.
- Weigh the person's hand with 3 to 5 kg until the shoulder is reduced.

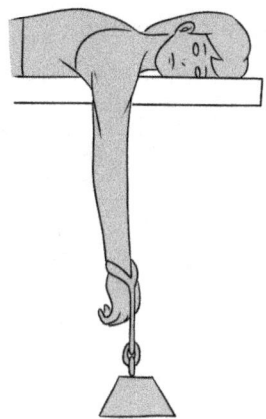

Patella Reduction

Gently straighten the patient's knee.

If the patella does not spontaneously reduce, gently guide it into position.

Splint the knee at about 10 degrees of flexion and stabilize the patella, e.g., tape, brace, etc.

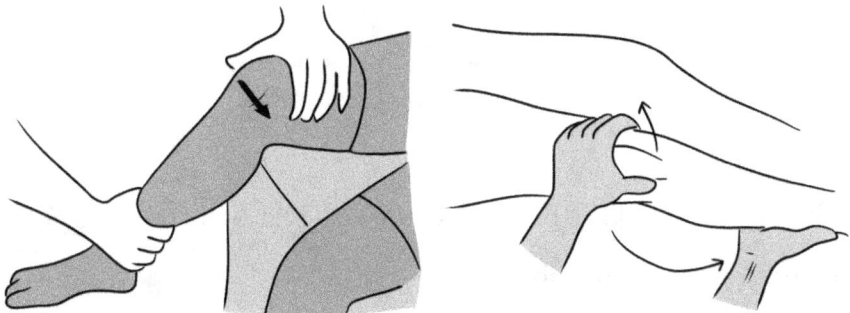

Digit Reduction

This includes fingers, thumbs, and toes.

Hold the finger/toe still near to the hand/foot. Pull out and traction into place.

Splint in its correct anatomical position.

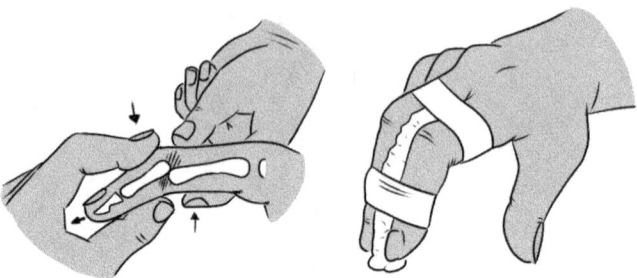

Ankle Reduction

An ankle dislocation usually comes with a fracture of one or both malleoli, i.e., the bony part on each side of the ankle.

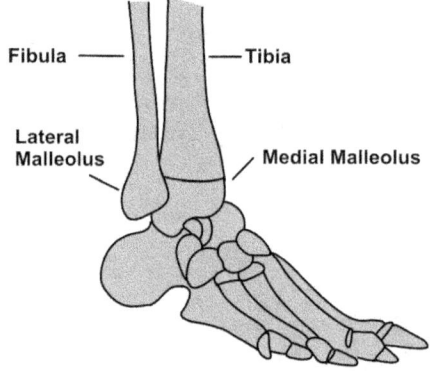

With the patient's knee bent, grasp the heel and apply traction.

Align the foot with the tibia.

Elbow Reduction

The patient keeps his/her elbow slightly flexed.

Apply counter-traction to hold the upper arm in place, e.g., using a second rescuer.

Apply traction of the lower arm out and down.

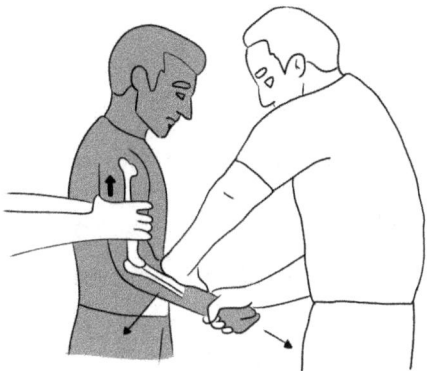

Wrist Reduction

Apply counter traction to hold the arm in place.

Grasp the fractured hand as if giving a handshake. Pull out with significant force.

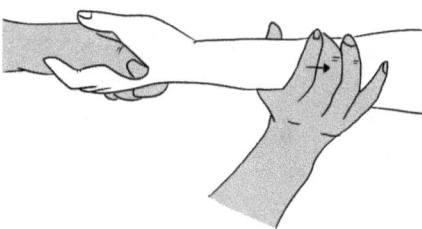

A downward movement may be needed.

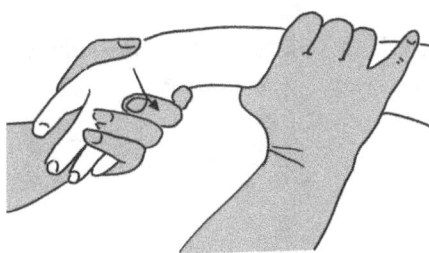

Hip Reduction

Place the patient on a flat, hard surface.

One rescuer stabilizes the pelvis by pushing down at/near the waist.

Bend the patient's knee.

Pull up and on the leg and, if possible, out on the thigh.

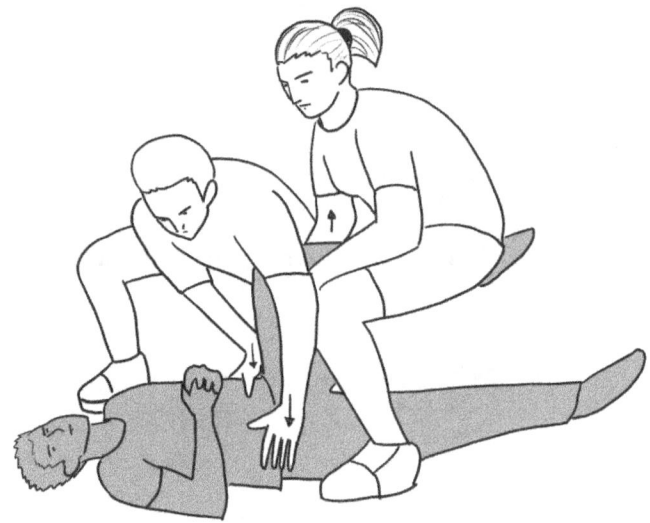

Related Chapters

- Diagnosis and Treatments > Musculoskeletal System > Musculoskeletal Injuries in General
- Diagnosis and Treatments > Musculoskeletal Injuries > Immobilization

FRACTURES

A fracture occurs when a bone is broken, most commonly due to trauma. All fractures are unstable injuries. Once immobilized, most fractures will take 6 to 8 weeks to heal (rejoin). Large-bone and complicated injuries may take longer.

For the purpose of this book, there are two main types of fractures: closed and open. A closed fracture occurs when there is a break in the bone but the skin is intact. An open fracture occurs when the skin is broken.

A closed fracture can become an open fracture if not treated well.

Symptoms of a Fracture

- Deep cut in the area of the injury (open fracture)
- Grinding sensation
- Inability to use the bone, i.e., patient cannot put any weight on it.
- Motion of the bone where there is no joint
- Severe pain, more so than a sprain
- Swelling and bruising, more so than a sprain

- In the case of your hand, a 'fifth knuckle'

Treatment for a Fracture

- Cut away clothing.
- If it is an open fracture, gently irrigate and dress.
- Check CSM.
- If CSM is compromised, reduction is needed.
- If CSM is okay, splint in place and seek advanced medical care.
- If there is no advanced medical care and the bone is deformed, reduction is needed in order for the bone to heal properly.

Notes:

- Reducing a fracture will be more painful and riskier than reducing a dislocation.
- Damage to nerves and blood vessels may occur.

Related Chapters

- Diagnosis and Treatments > Musculoskeletal System > Musculoskeletal Injuries in General
- Diagnosis and Treatments > Musculoskeletal System > Dislocations > Reductions
- Diagnosis and Treatments > Musculoskeletal System > Sprains and Strains > Sprains

FRACTURED RIBS

Fractured ribs usually occur along the side of the chest. Pushing on the sternum will produce pain at the site of the fracture.

Symptoms of Fractured Ribs

- Pain in the chest after blunt chest trauma
- Pain when breathing

Treatment for Fractured Ribs

Treat flail chest if applicable (below); otherwise:

- Do not tape the ribs.
- Encourage deep breathing at least 10 times per hour.
- Position of comfort.
- Monitor and treat for pneumothorax (punctured lung) if needed.
- Transport injured side down.

Related Chapters

- Diagnosis and Treatment > Musculoskeletal System > Pneumothorax

FLAIL CHEST

Flail chest occurs when a part of the rib cage breaks away from the chest wall, i.e., when three or more ribs are broken in two or more places due to blunt trauma.

Symptoms of a Flail Chest

- Extreme chest pain
- Impaired breathing
- Visual sign of the chest wall moving in and out when breathing

Treatment for a Flail Chest

- Pad heavily, e.g., rolled-up clothing (use hand pressure to keep it on).
- Roll patient onto flail side if possible.
- Monitor for pneumothorax.
- Seek advanced medical treatment.

Related Chapters

- Diagnosis and Treatments > Musculoskeletal System > Pneumothorax

FRACTURED PELVIS

A fractured pelvis is extremely painful and can result in major blood loss.

Symptoms of a Fractured Pelvis

- Bruising and pain around the pelvis
- Impaired CSM

Treatment for a Fractured Pelvis

- A pelvic sling can be improvised with such things as clothes, a sleeping bag, sleeping mat, tent, etc.
- The aim is to achieve circumferential binding.
- Remove any object that may cause discomfort, e.g., belt, pocket items.
- Slide the sling under the bony part of the hips and cross it over the front of the pelvis.
- Apply so the pressure is focused over the greater trochanter of the femur (the part of the femur connecting it to the hip bone).
- Tighten enough for stabilization and comfort.

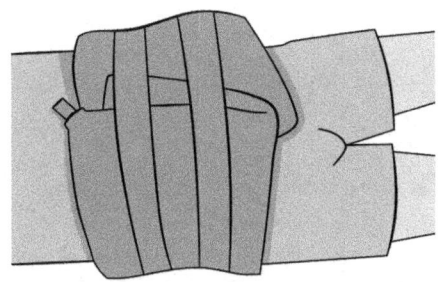

Related Chapters

- Diagnosis and Treatments > Musculoskeletal System > Musculoskeletal Injuries in General

SPRAINS AND STRAINS

SPRAINS

A sprain occurs when a ligament (the fibrous tissue that connects one bone to another) is excessively stretched due to the forcing of a joint beyond its normal range of motion.

A twisted ankle is a common type of sprain.

Symptoms of Sprains

- Bruising
- Pain
- Swelling

Treatment for Sprains

Most sprains will heal over time. Severe knee sprains may require surgery to heal completely.

- RICES
- Immobilize if unstable
- Anti-inflammatory

Related Chapters

- Diagnosis and Treatments > Musculoskeletal System > Musculoskeletal Injuries in General
- Diagnosis and Treatments > Musculoskeletal System > Immobilization

STRAINS

Strains occur when the muscle or its tendon (tissue that connects the muscle to connect to bone) is partially torn. Back muscles are most commonly strained.

Daily morning stretches and correct lifting techniques will help prevent strains.

Correct Lifting Techniques

- Don't lift things while unbalanced.
- Don't reach for an object, i.e., hold it as close to your body as possible when lifting.
- Don't twist while lifting.
- Lift with your legs and a straight back.
- If carrying a pack, keep the weight of it on your hips as opposed to your shoulders.

Treatment for Strains

- Mild massage
- Anti-inflammatory
- Muscle relaxer
- Ginger and raw honey tea
- Salicin poultice

RESPIRATORY SYSTEM

ASTHMA

When a person with asthma is exposed to a substance that they are allergic to (allergen), their airway can swell, which decreases the amount of air that can get to the lungs. This is known as an asthma attack.

There are a variety of triggers depending on the sufferer. Some common ones are animal hair, cold air, dust and dust mites, infection, mold and mildew, overexertion, pollen, pollutants, severe stress, smoke, various medicines, etc.

Symptoms of an Asthma Attack

Symptoms vary from attack to attack and from individual to individual.

Mild:

- Agitation
- Increased respiratory rate
- Moderate wheezing at end of each breath
- Pulse under 100 bpm
- Shortness of breath while walking

Moderate:

- Agitation
- Loud wheezing
- Patient prefers to sit.
- Pulse 100 to 120 bpm
- Shortness of breath while talking
- Talking in short phrases
- Use of accessory muscles (shoulder girdle and chest wall) when breathing

Severe:

- Agitation
- Cyanosis (blue, gray, or purple coloration of the skin; usually lips, fingertips, and/or face)
- Confusion
- Drowsiness
- Higher-pitched wheezing
- Lung sounds may be loud or diminished.
- Pulse over 120 bpm
- Respiratory rate greater than 30 bpm
- Shortness of breath while resting
- Patient sits upright.
- Patient talks in one-to-two-word sentences.
- Unconsciousness

Treatment for an Asthma Attack

When treating asthma, the main idea is to avoid the cause and to maintain an open airway.

In mild to moderate cases, patients will often know what to do and can treat themselves.

- Minimize the causes.
- Albuterol: Two puffs and rest will usually do the trick. An increased heart rate is a common side effect.
- If patients do not respond to their self-medication and/or severe symptoms are present, the following action can be taken:
- PROP
- Epinephrine if needed: 0.01 ml/kg of body weight, maximum dose of 0.3 ml; injections can be repeated every 5 minutes if needed.
- Corticosteroid: Prednisone 1 mg/kg of body weight, maximum dose of 60 mg once a day.

- Albuterol or the patient's equivalent, 6 to 10 puffs which can be repeated every 20 minutes for up to 3 doses.
- Seek advanced medical care.

Alternative remedies may be effective in mild to moderate cases.

- Herbal teas: Chamomile, ginger and garlic, nettle, rosemary
- Coffee: Black unsweetened coffee
- Honey: Breathe deeply from a jar of honey for quick relief.

Prevention of Asthma Attacks

- Honey: Drink raw honey tea a few times a day.
- Stay away from known allergens and other triggers.
- Diet control: Avoid dairy, eat organic, hydrate well, increase intake of omega-3 fatty acids, and replace animal proteins with plant proteins.
- Breathing methods: Activities such as swimming, yoga, meditation, etc., can help to regulate and improve breathing habits.

Dirgha pranayama (three-part breath) is a yoga breathing exercise:

- Sit in a comfortable cross-legged position and don't slouch.
- Relax your abdomen.
- Place your palms on your belly.
- Breathe deeply into your lower lungs, feeling your belly expand.
- Repeat this breath three to four times.
- Next, place your palms on the sides of your rib cage.
- Breathe into your chest, feeling your rib cage expand.
- Repeat this breath three to four times.
- Now, place your fingertips on the front of your chest just below your collarbones.

- Breathe into the upper part of your chest and feel your hands lifting.
- Repeat this breath three to four times.
- Finally, combine all three in-breaths.
- Exhale completely and gently squeeze your abdomen to expel all the air.
- Repeat the whole cycle three to four times.
- Focus on filling and emptying your lungs completely.

Related Chapters

- Must Read > Immediate First Aid > Critical First Aid > Breathing

BRONCHITIS

Bronchitis is an inflammation of the tubes that carry air to your lungs (the bronchial tubes). If left untreated, it may lead to pneumonia.

There are two main types of bronchitis:

Acute bronchitis is common and usually stems from another respiratory infection, e.g., common cold. It will usually only last a few days, although the cough may linger for weeks.

Chronic bronchitis is more serious and requires advanced medical care. Smoking is the most common cause, but dust, pollution, toxic gases, etc., may also cause the condition.

Symptoms of Bronchitis

- Chest tightness
- Cough producing mucus
- Fatigue
- Mild fever and chills
- Shortness of breath
- Wheezing

The difference in symptoms between acute and chronic bronchitis is as follows:

Acute bronchitis will resolve quickly although a nagging cough may persist for several weeks.

Chronic bronchitis will involve a productive cough for at least three months and will reoccur.

Treatment for Bronchitis

- Avoid irritants (fumes, smoke, etc.).

- Hydrate.
- Rest.
- If chronic bronchitis is suspected, seek advanced medical care.
- Antibiotic: Amoxicillin-clavulanate 875 mg every 12 hours for 7 to 10 days.
- Antibiotic: Ciprofloxacin 500 mg every 12 hours for 7 to 14 days, or 750 mg every 12 hours for 7 to 14 days for severe cases.
- Antibiotic: Doxycycline 200 mg on the first day given in 2 doses, followed by 100 mg per day, or 100 mg every 12 hours for severe cases.
- Antibiotics, other: Amoxicillin, ampicillin, azithromycin, levofloxacin, sulfamethoxazole/trimethoprim, tetracycline
- Cough suppressant: Not for chronic bronchitis

Related Chapters

- Diagnosis and Treatments > Respiratory System > Pneumonia

COLD AND FLU

The common cold and influenza are both respiratory infections. Technically they are different, but for practical purposes, and because initial treatment is the same, the flu can be considered a more serious cold.

The common flu can be countered with a yearly vaccination. Special precautions must be taken if in threat of more serious strains of influenza, e.g., swine flu, bird flu.

Caution: Meningitis is a potentially deadly virus that has very similar symptoms to influenza.

Symptoms of Cold and Flu

Symptom	Influenza	Cold
Symptom onset	3 to 6 hours	Gradually
Aches	Usual, often severe	Slight
Chest discomfort	Often severe	Mild to moderate
Chills	Fairly common	Uncommon
Coughing	Dry, unproductive	Hacking, productive cough
Fever	Usually present	Rare
Headache	Common	Uncommon
Sneezing	Uncommon	Common
Sore throat	Uncommon	Common
Stuffy nose	Uncommon	Common
Tiredness	Moderate to severe	Mild

Treatment for Cold and Flu

Basic treatment for cold and minor flu is the same. Flu will probably take a week or two until complete recovery, whereas a cold may only take a few days.

- Treat symptoms, e.g., throat lozenges, pain and fever meds, decongestants.
- Avoid alcohol, cigarettes, and recreational drugs.
- Avoid flying.
- Hot or cold packs around your congested sinuses
- Hydration with hot clear fluids, e.g., soup, water
- Rest
- Steam inhalation and/or steamy showers
- Antiviral: Tamiflu 75 mg twice a day for 5 days.

If taken early enough, Tamiflu may completely prevent the flu, but if not taken within the first 48 hours of symptoms, it won't have much effect at all.

- Garlic, ginger, and honey tea: 3 cups a day (acts as a cough syrup and will ease a sore throat).
- Salicin tea
- Water and vinegar sponge baths (combats fever)

Seek advanced medical care and consider antiviral medication for more serious bouts of flu with any of the following symptoms:

- Altered skin color, i.e., grayish or bluish
- Confusion
- Flu-like symptoms that improve but then return with fever and cough
- High fever for more than 3 days
- Hyperventilation
- Respiratory distress

- Pain or pressure in the chest or abdomen
- Severe vomiting
- Sudden dizziness

Related Chapters

- Diagnosis and Treatments > Head > Brain > Meningitis

DRY COUGH

A cough can be a symptom in many cases, but sometimes it is also just a dry cough due to altitude, dry air, irritants, etc.

If it produces phlegm, blood, etc., or comes with other symptoms, e.g., fever, then it is more than just a cough and the underlying cause should be treated accordingly.

Treatment for a Dry Cough

- Cough suppressants at night
- Throat lozenges

PNEUMONIA

Pneumonia is a disease of the lungs that often results from a lung infection. Lots of things can cause pneumonia including bacteria, chemicals, viruses, fungi, other infectious agents, etc.

Symptoms of Pneumonia

- Chest cold
- Chest pain
- Chills
- Coughing up different colors of mycous
- Fever
- Mild fever, less than 38.5 °C (102 °F)
- Muscle aches
- Productive cough
- Tiredness
- Wheezing
- Weakness

Treatment for Pneumonia

- Hydration
- Pain/fever meds
- Rest
- Antibiotic: Amoxicillin-clavulanate 875 mg every 12 hours for 7 to 10 days in the case of pneumococcal pneumonia, or up to 21 days for other.
- Antibiotic: Doxycycline 200 mg on the first day given in 2 divided doses followed by 100 mg a day, or 100 mg every 12 hours for severe cases.
- Antibiotics, other: Amoxicillin, ampicillin, azithromycin, levofloxacin, metronidazole, sulfamethoxazole/trimethoprim, tetracycline

When to seek advanced medical care:

- Coughing up blood
- Excessive vomiting
- Shortness of breath, either at rest or with just a little exertion
- Severe chest pain
- Severe weakness

For serious bouts of pneumonia where no medical drugs are available, it is important to keep the patient interested and on his/her feet. Do not let them "give up in a corner."

SORE THROAT

A sore throat is a common symptom for many ailments and also presents its own problems, e.g., difficulty swallowing, pain.

If there are red or white blotches in the back of the mouth, it may be pharyngitis (throat infection), e.g., strep throat.

Treatment for a Sore Throat

- Gargle warm salt water.
- Anti-inflammatory
- Lozenges
- Garlic, ginger, honey and lemon tea(s)
- Salicin tea

Related Chapters

- Diagnosis and Treatments > Respiratory System > Strep Throat

STREP THROAT

Strep throat (streptococcal pharyngitis) is a contagious bacterial throat infection spread via close contact with an infected host. If untreated, it may lead to kidney inflammation or rheumatic fever.

Symptoms of Strep Throat

- Fatigue
- Fever
- Headache
- Rash
- Small white spots on the back of the throat and/or tonsils
- Sore throat
- Stomachache
- Swollen tonsils
- Tiny red spots at the back of the roof of the mouth
- Vomiting

Treatment for Strep Throat

- Rest and hydration
- Treatment of symptoms
- Antibiotic: Amoxicillin/clavulanate 500 mg every 12 hours for 10 days, or 875 mg every 12 hours in severe cases.
- Antibiotic: Doxycycline 200 mg on the first day given in 2 evenly divided doses followed by 100 mg per day, or 100 mg every 12 hours in severe cases.
- Antibiotics, other: Amoxicillin, ampicillin, azithromycin, cephalexin, sulfamethoxazole/trimethoprim, tetracycline

Symptoms usually subside after 48 hours of antibiotic treatment, but finish the whole course.

WHOOPING COUGH

Whooping cough (pertussis) is a highly contagious bacterial infection. It is most common in unimmunized infants and teenagers whose immunity has started to fade. Vaccines are available.

Symptoms of Whooping Cough

Symptoms come in three stages.

Stage 1 usually lasts for 1 to 2 weeks and mimics the common cold:

- Cough (mild)
- Fever (mild)
- Nasal congestion
- Runny nose
- Sneezing
- Red, watery eyes

Stage 2 usually lasts 2 to 4 weeks and is characterized by severe, uncontrollable coughing which may cause:

- Extreme fatigue.
- Red or blue face.
- Vomiting.
- Whooping sound on inhale (mainly in children).

Stage 3 is the recovery phase. This is characterized by a gradual easing of symptoms which may last for months.

Treatment for Whooping Cough

- Cool-mist vaporizer
- Hydrate.
- Remove irritants, e.g., aerosols, smoke.

- Rest
- Smaller, more frequent meals (prevents vomiting)
- Patients should cover their cough and wash hands often.
- People in contact with patients should wear a mask.
- Cough medicine will probably not help.
- Antibiotic: Amoxicillin/clavulanate 500 mg every 12 hours for 10 days, or 875 mg every 12 hours for severe cases.
- Antibiotic: Doxycycline 200 mg on the first day given in 2 doses followed by 100 mg per day, or 100 mg every 12 hours for severe cases.
- Antibiotics, other: Amoxicillin, ampicillin, azithromycin, cephalexin, sulfamethoxazole/trimethoprim, tetracycline

THANKS FOR READING

Dear reader,

Thank you for reading *Wilderness And Travel Medicine*.

If you enjoyed this book, please leave a review where you bought it. It helps more than most people think.

Don't forget your FREE book chapters!

You will also be among the first to know of FREE review copies, discount offers, bonus content, and more.

Go to:

https://offers.SFNonfictionBooks.com/Free-Chapters

Thanks again for your support.

REFERENCES

Alton, J. (2016). *The Survival Medicine Handbook.* Doom and Bloom.

Auerbach, P. Constance, B Freer, L. (2018). *Field Guide to Wilderness Medicine.* Elsevier.

Fiedler, C. (2009). *The Complete Idiot's Guide to Natural Remedies.* Alpha.

Hawke, M. Hawke, R. (2018). *Family Survival Guide.* Skyhorse.

Miller, T. (2012). *Beyond Collapse.* CreateSpace Independent Publishing Platform.

Morris, B. (2019). *The Green Beret Survival Guide.* Skyhorse.

WA Police, SA. (2019). *Aids to Survival.*

Wiseman, J. (2015). *SAS Survival Guide.* William Collins.

AUTHOR RECOMMENDATIONS

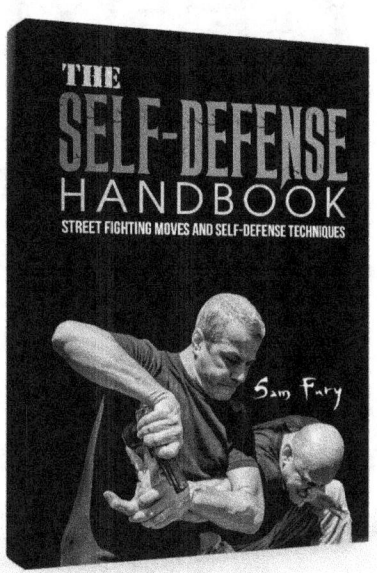

Teach Yourself Self-Defense

This is the only self-defense training manual you need, because these are the best street fighting moves around.

Get it now.

www.SFNonfictionBooks.com/Self-Defense-Handbook

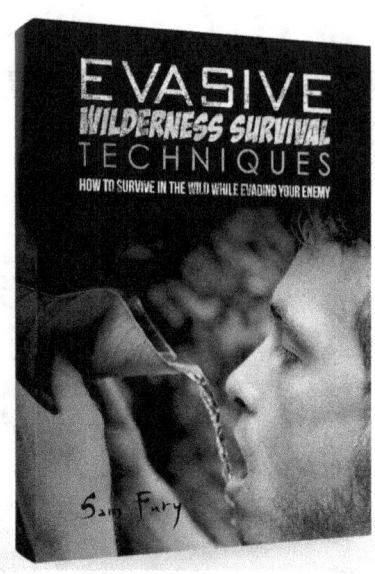

Teach Yourself Evasive Wilderness Survival

Discover all the evasive survival skills you need, because if you can survive under these circumstances, you can survive anything.

Get it now.

www.SFNonfictionBooks.com/Evasive-Wilderness-Survival-Techniques

ABOUT SAM FURY

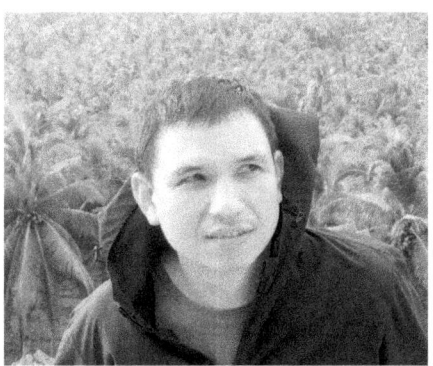

Sam Fury has had a passion for survival, evasion, resistance, and escape (SERE) training since he was a young boy growing up in Australia.

This led him to years of training and career experience in related subjects, including martial arts, military training, survival skills, outdoor sports, and sustainable living.

These days, Sam spends his time refining existing skills, gaining new skills, and sharing what he learns via the Survival Fitness Plan website.

www.SurvivalFitnessPlan.com

- amazon.com/author/samfury
- goodreads.com/SamFury
- facebook.com/AuthorSamFury
- instagram.com/AuthorSamFury
- youtube.com/SurvivalFitnessPlan

www.ingramcontent.com/pod-product-compliance
Lightning Source LLC
Chambersburg PA
CBHW071113080526
44587CB00013B/1326